MEDICAL RESEARCH WRITING MADE EASY

MEDICAL RESEARCH WRITING MADE EASY

Dr. Vinoth Gnana Chellaiyan

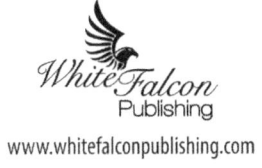

WhiteFalcon
Publishing
www.whitefalconpublishing.com

Medical Research Writing Made Easy
Vinoth Gnana Chellaiyan

www.whitefalconpublishing.com

Requests for permission should be addressed to
drchellaiyan@gmail.com

ISBN - 978-1-63640-587-2

CONTENTS

PREFACE

Greetings!

This book is intended to assist students, faculty, and researchers in the early stages of their research careers. It is recommended that readers read the chapters from beginning to end in order to get the most out of this book. Practice all of the assignments and make an effort to comprehend all of the examples provided.

One of the book's distinguishing features is that it discusses the structuring of a phrase – the use of nouns, verbs, voice, prepositions, and sentence structure – which could be very useful for researchers who are just starting out. The chapter on writing original articles covered several aspects, such as table and figure construction, abstract writing, discussion and conclusion writing. Peer review, plagiarism, and publication in medical journals are hot topics.

The protocol writing topic is comprehensive and would be useful for students and researchers who submit proposals to ethics and research committees, as well as for grant submission. The book contains numerous examples that will help the reader understand the various topics and master the art of scientific writing.

Above all, writing this book would not have been possible without the Almighty's blessings.

I wish you the best of luck in your research career.

– Dr DVG Chellaiyan

DISCLAIMER

This book is a simple guide for medical students, faculty, and researchers. Many of the examples used in this book are solely for illustration purposes.

1

GETTING STARTED

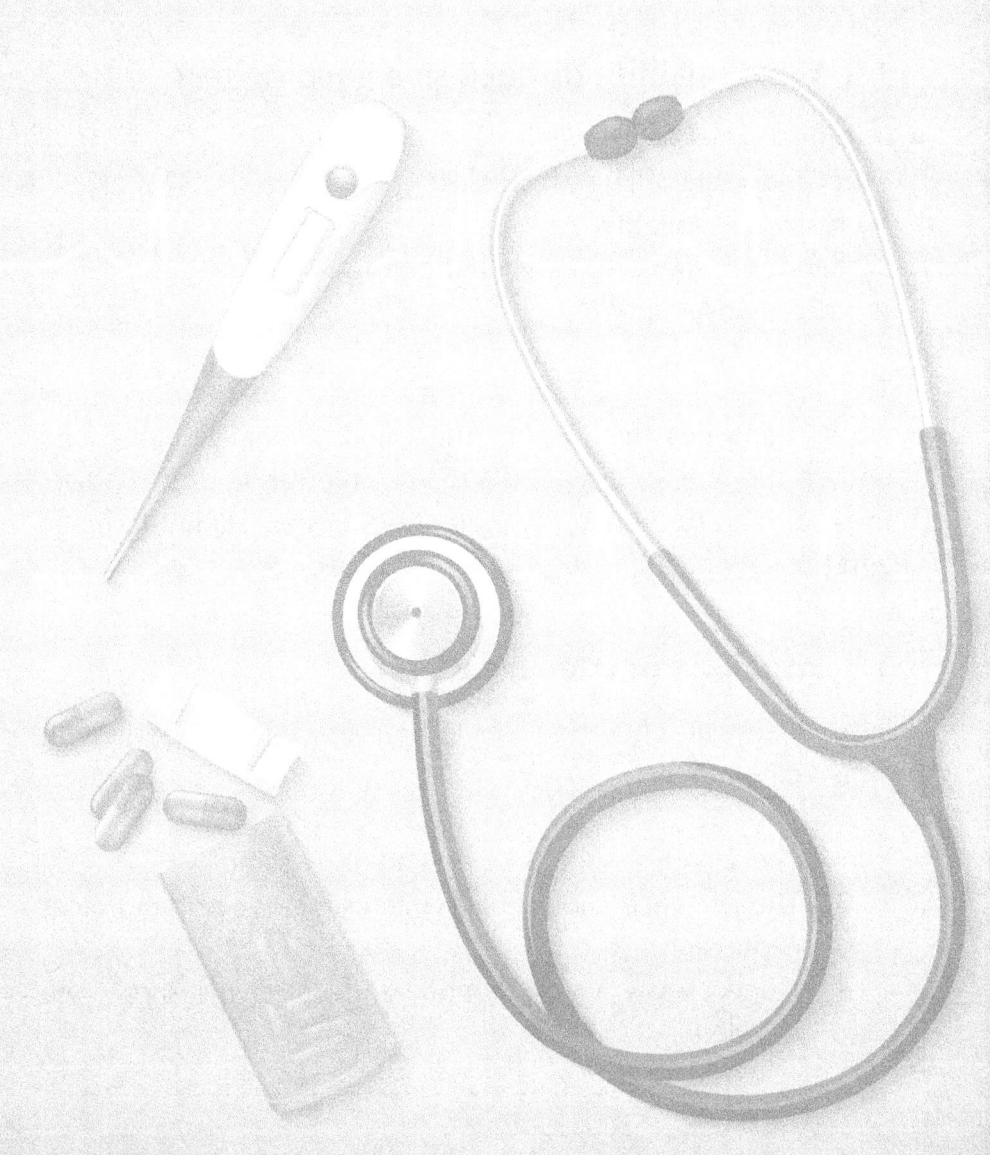

1.1 What makes good writing?

Good writing is very essential for the readers to understand what we intend to convey. Clear and effective communication of an idea is achieved through good writing. The clear idea that we have in our minds needs to be translated into sentences. In addition, good writing is elegant and stylish. To achieve this, it takes time, revision, and a good editor!

1.2 What qualities distinguish a good writer?

Is it innate talent?
Years and years of English classes?
A creative personality?
What are the effects of alcohol and drugs?
Is it divine inspiration?

The answer is no. Good writing can be learned! A good writer translates the idea in the mind into a valuable and understandable phrase and creates interest in the reader's mind to read further. A competent writer has a point to make and thinks logically.

1.3 Principles of effective writing

Listed below are the principles to be followed while writing in a medical journal:

1. The sentence should be easy to understand.
2. The sentence should have interesting content and clear expression.
3. Unnecessary words, jargon, and acronyms should be avoided.

4. The sentence should have the correct voice.

5. Usage of verbs and nouns should be appropriate.

The following examples contain a few sentences taken from various articles published in medical journals.

Example 1:

Adoptive cell transfer (ACT) immunotherapy is based on the ex vivo selection of tumor-reactive lymphocytes, and their activation and numerical expression before reinfusion to the autologous tumor-bearing host.

(Ref: Dudley ME et al. Adoptive cell transfer therapy following non-myeloablative but lymphodepleting chemotherapy for the treatment of patients with refractory metastatic melanoma. J Clin Oncol. 2005 Apr 1;23(10):2346-57)

- Is this sentence simple to grasp?
- Is it enjoyable and interesting to read this sentence?

Answer:

In the example cited above, the sentences may seem fine, but there are some issues to be addressed. Spunky verbs were transformed into clunky nouns, which is a common practice in academic writing.

These words are highlighted below:

Adoptive cell transfer (ACT) immunotherapy is based on the ex vivo **selection** of tumor-reactive lymphocytes, and their **activation** and numerical **expression** before **reinfusion** to the autologous tumor-bearing host.

Rewriting attempt:

Adoptive cell transfer (ACT) immunotherapy is done by selecting and activating tumor-reactive lymphocytes ex vivo. This is followed by expressing and reinfusing to the autologous tumor-bearing host.

Example 3:

Dysregulation of physiologic microRNA (miR) activity has been shown to play an important role in tumor initiation and progression, including gliomagenesis. Therefore, molecular species that can regulate miR activity on their target RNAs without affecting the expression of relevant mature miRs may play equally relevant roles in cancer.

(Ref: Sumazin P et al. An extensive microRNA-mediated network of RNA-RNA interactions regulates established oncogenic pathways in glioblastoma. Cell. 2011 Oct 14;147(2):370-81)

Is this sentence readable and understandable easily?

Answer:

There are four elements to consider in this statement - nouns, words, jargon, and voice.

1. Take note of the use of nouns rather than verbs.
   Dysregulation of physiologic microRNA (miR) activity has been shown to play an important role in tumor **initiation** and **progression**, including gliomagenesis. Therefore, molecular species that can regulate miR activity on their target RNAs without affecting the **expression** of relevant mature miRs may play equally relevant roles in cancer.

2. Take note of the use of ambiguous terminology
   Dysregulation of **physiologic** microRNA (miR) activity has been shown to play an important role in tumor initiation and progression, including gliomagenesis. Therefore, **molecular species** that can regulate miR activity on their target RNAs without affecting the expression of relevant mature miRs may play equally relevant roles in cancer.

3. Take note of the overuse of jargon and acronyms.
   Dysregulation of physiologic **microRNA (miR)** activity has been shown to play an important role in tumor initiation and progression, including <u>gliomagenesis</u>. Therefore, molecular species that can regulate <u>miR</u> activity on their target RNAs without affecting the expression of relevant mature <u>miRs</u> may play equally relevant roles in cancer.

4. Take note of the passive voice.
   Dysregulation of physiologic microRNA (miR) activity **has been shown** to play an important role in tumor initiation and progression, including gliomagenesis. Therefore, molecular species that can regulate miR activity on their target RNAs without affecting the expression of relevant mature miRs may play equally relevant roles in cancer.

5. In addition, note the distance between the subject and the main verb of this sentence.
   Dysregulation of physiologic microRNA (miR) activity has been shown to play an important role in tumor initiation and progression, including gliomagenesis. Therefore, **molecular species** that can regulate miR activity on their target RNAs without affecting the expression of relevant mature miRs **may play** equally relevant roles in cancer.

Possible rewrite:

Changes in microRNA expression play a role in cancer, including glioma. Therefore, events that disrupt microRNAs from binding to their target RNAs may also promote cancer.

Nuggets

Complex ideas do not necessitate the use of complicated language. Scientific writing should be simple to read, if not enjoyable!

1.4 Attention while using acronyms

An acronym is a word formed by combining the first letters of each word in a group of words. Some people distinguish between a word-like acronym (such as NATO) and an initialism (such as FBI), in which each letter is pronounced separately.

The majority of people, on the other hand, are completely oblivious to such disparities. In scientific writing, acronyms are used to speed up the reading process and make the content of a document easier to understand. As a result, the purpose of acronym use is usually for the abbreviation to be well-known, to save a lot of space, and/or to avoid tedious repetition.

1.5 Steps in becoming a better writer:

The following steps may be followed to improve our output of writing:

- Read medical journals, pay attention, and try to imitate the writing.
- Experiment with writing for medical journals and medical news.

- Abandon regular 'academic' writing habits (this is a deprogramming step!)
- Master the art of ruthless cutting. Never let your words become too attached to you.
- Before you try to write about your research, discuss about it.
- Instead of boring your readers, write to engage them!
- Go over everything again. Nobody gets everything right on the first try.
- Hire a good editor to polish and copyedit your work.
- Take chances.

2

PRINCIPLES OF EFFECTIVE WRITING

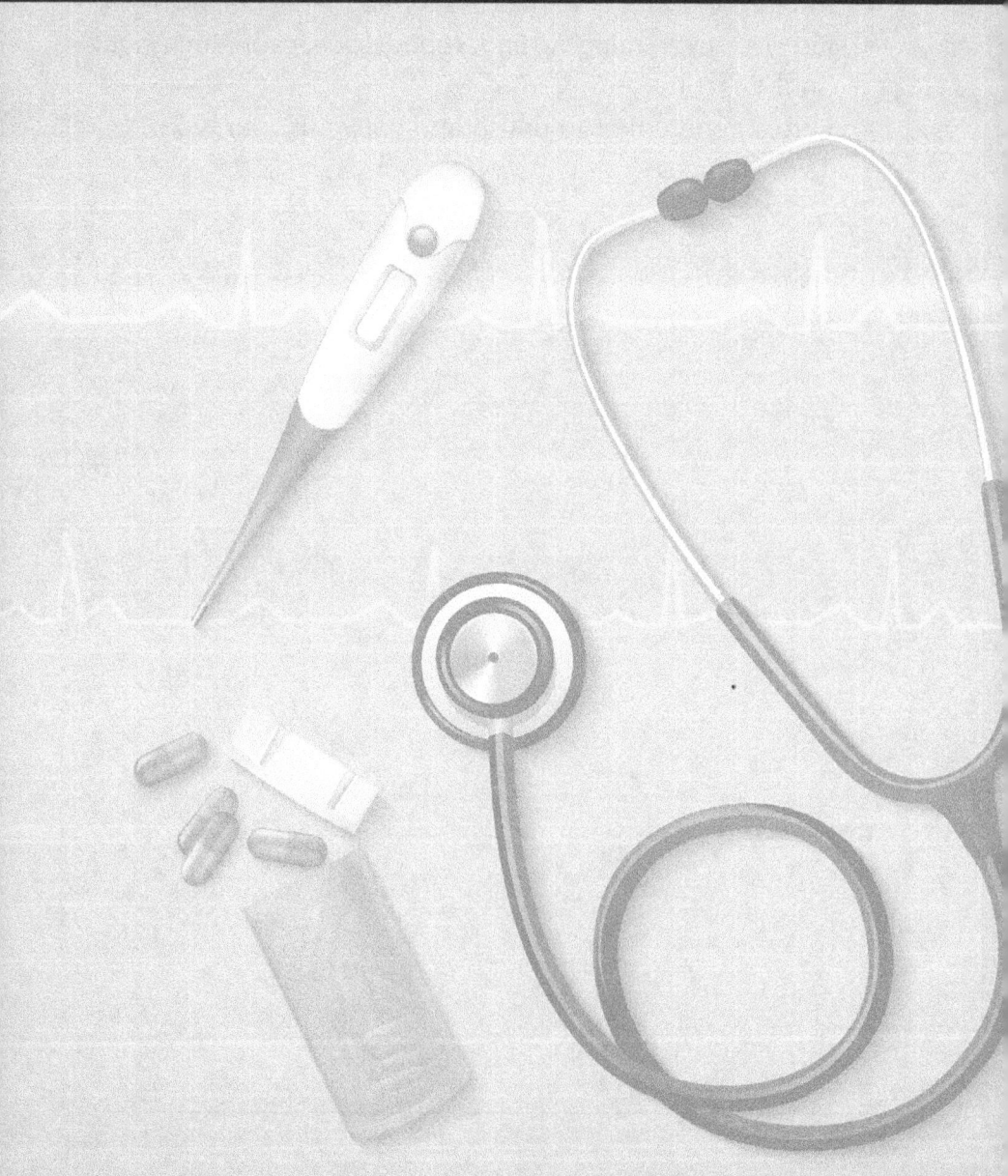

"The secret of good writing is to strip every sentence to its cleanest components. Every word that serves no function, every long word that could be a short word, every adverb that carries the same meaning that's already in the verb, every passive construction that leaves the reader unsure of who is doing what—these are the thousand and one adulterants that weaken the strength of a sentence. And they usually occur in proportion to the education and rank."

-William Zinsser in On Writing Well, 1976

2.1 Cut the clutter

Decluttering the paragraph or cutting the clutter makes the sentences more interesting to the readers.

Example 1:

This paper provides a review of the basic principles of cancer biology study design, using as examples studies that illustrate the methodologic challenges or that demonstrate successful solutions to the difficulties inherent in biological research.

Rewrite:

> This paper reviews cancer biology study design, using examples that illustrate specific challenges and solutions.

Example 2:

As it is well known, increased athletic activity has been related to a profile of lower cardiovascular risk, lower blood pressure levels, and improved muscular and cardio-respiratory performance.

Rewrite:

Increased athletic activity is associated with lower cardiovascular risk, lower blood pressure, and improved fitness.

2.2 Common clutters

Following is a list of common clutters that we use regularly in writing but could be avoided.

1. Deadweight phrases and words
   a. As it is clear
   b. As it has been demonstrated
   c. It can be stated that
   d. It should be emphasized that
2. Vague words and phrases
   a. Fundamental of
   b. methodologic
   c. significant
3. Long words or phrases
   a. cardiorespiratory and muscular performance
4. Unnecessary jargon and acronyms
   a. miR
   b. Gliomagenesis
   c. muscular and cardiorespiratory performance
5. Repetitive phrases or words
   a. difficulties/challenges
   b. illustrate/demonstrate
   c. successful solutions
   d. studies/examples
   e. adverbs
   f. very, quite, basically, really, generally, etc.

2.3 Cutting Extra Words

In cutting down the extra words, be observant and ruthless. We often find it difficult to let go of words after putting so much effort into them. However, resist their enticing pull. Try framing the sentence without the filler words to see how much more effectively it conveys the very same idea.

Example 1:

Hodgkin's Lymphoma incidence shows two peak periods in most of the published literature: rates are the highest in both young and the elderly population.

Rewrite:

Hodgkin's Lymphoma peaks in the young and the elderly.

2.4 Long words and phrases

Long words and phrases could be made short.

Table 2.1 List of long phrases with shorter alternatives

Wordy version	Crisp version
Have an effect on	Affect
A majority of	Most
Due to the fact that	Because
Give rise to	Cause
Less frequently occurring	Rare
Are of the same opinion	Agree
A number of	Many
All three of the	Three

Example 1:

Based on the assumption that intelligence is normally distributed, the expected prevalence of intellectual disability is around 2%.

Rewrite:

> The expected prevalence of intellectual disability, if intelligence is normally distributed, is 2%.

2.5 Repetitive Words or Clauses

It happens to most of us. Words that we use frequently are likely to hang out in our subconscious. And some linger longer than others, eventually finding their way into our writing through the natural flow of words.

Consider the following tips to avoid sounding like a broken record.

2.5.1 Change the wording

Example 1:

A strong cell-mediated immune response is essential, and deficiency in this response predisposes an individual towards active TB.

Rewrite:

> Deficiency in T-cell-mediated immune response predisposes an individual to active TB.

2.5.2 Eliminate negatives

Example 1:

She was not often right in orientation to time.

Rewrite:

She was usually wrong in orientation to time.

Example 2:

The trial found that the drug was harmful.

Rewrite:

The trial found the drug safe.

Table 2.2 List of regular negatives with better alternatives

Regular negatives	Better words
Does not have	Lacks
Not harmful	Safe
Did not succeed	Failed
Not honest	Dishonest
Did not concentrate/pay attention to	Ignored
Did not remember	Forgot
Not important	Unimportant

2.5.3 Eliminate "There are"/"There is"

Example 1:

There was a straight line of bacterial growth on the agar plate.

Rewrite:

Bacterial growth lined the agar plate.

Example 2:

The research study confirmed that there is an association between alcohol and cancer.

Rewrite:

> The research study confirmed an association between alcohol and cancer.

2.5.4 Remove superfluous prepositions

For example, the words "that" and "on" are often unnecessary.

Example 1:

The infection occurred on 3rd day after surgery.

Rewrite:

> The infection occurred 3rd day after surgery.

Example 2:

They agreed that it was true.

Rewrite:

> They agreed it was true.

2.6 Points to Remember

Consider the following suggestions to reduce clutter in your writing:

1. Convert long clauses into shorter phrases.
2. Condense phrases into single words.
3. Avoid the sentence openers "There is", "There are", and "There were".
4. Avoid overusing modifiers.

5. Avoid duplication.
6. Employ active verbs.
7. Don't try to brag.
8. Remove any unnecessary phrases.
9. Avoid using verbs in noun forms.
10. Substitute more specific words for vague nouns.

Nuggets

- Remove superfluous words and phrases; learn to let go of your words!

- Use the active voice (subject + verb + object) to express yourself.

- Use strong verbs, avoid turning verbs into nouns, and don't bury the main verb!

2.10 Assessment

Questions:

1. Anti-inflammatory drugs may be protective for the occurrence of Alzheimer's disease.
2. Clinical seizures have been estimated to occur in 0.5% to 2.3% of the neonatal population.

Answers:

1. Anti-inflammatory drugs may protect against Alzheimer's disease.
2. Clinical seizures occur in 0.5% to 2.3% of newborns.

3

THE ART OF WRITING - HANDLING VERBS AND NOUNS

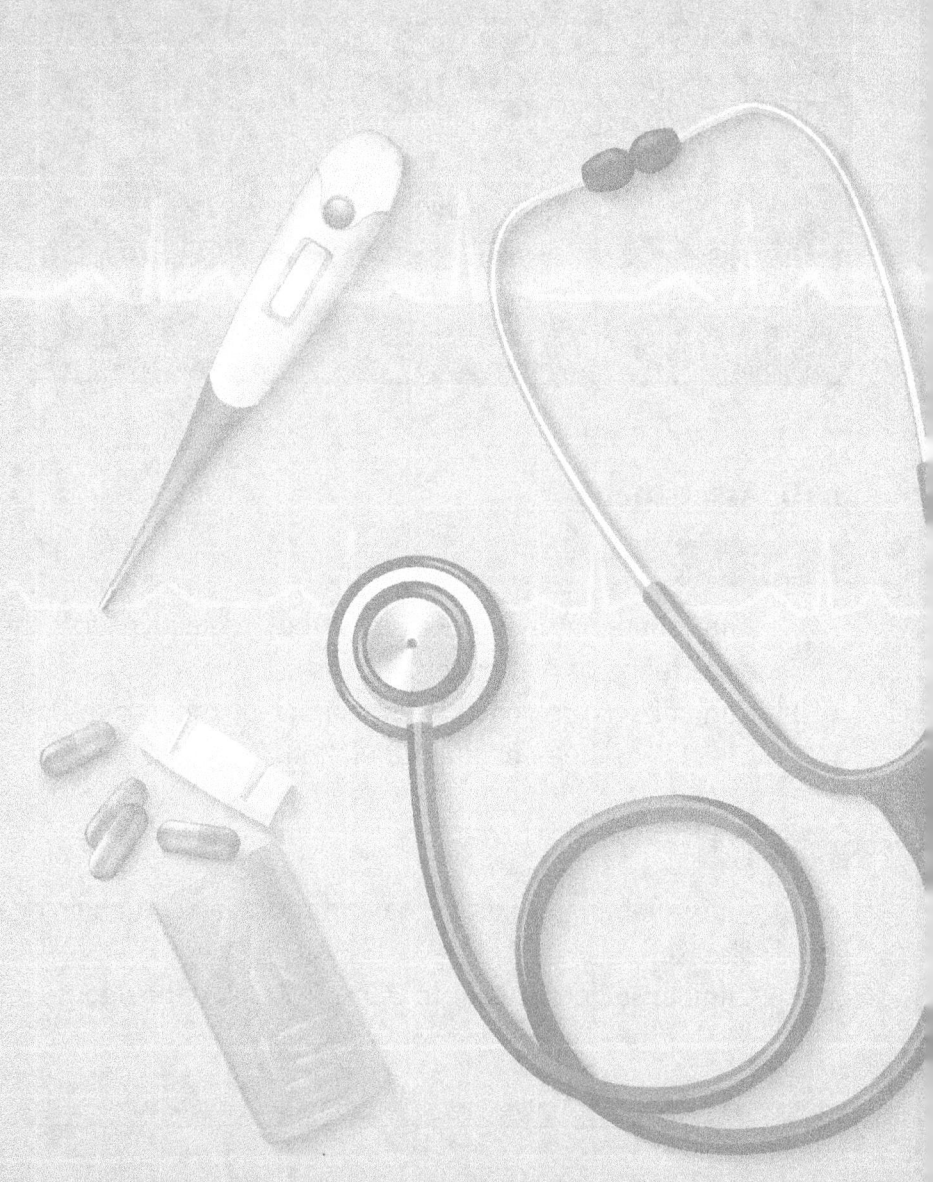

3.1 Parts of a Sentence

The subject, verb, and (often, but not always) object are the three basic components of a sentence. Typically, the subject is a noun — a word that refers to a person, place, or thing. The verb (or predicate) usually comes after the subject and refers to an action or state of being. The action is received by an object, which usually follows the verb. The two grammatical voices are active and passive. The form of a verb that indicates when a subject acts or is the receiver of an action is referred to as the voice. When the subject performs the action, the voice is active, and when the subject receives the action, the voice is passive.

3.2 Voices

Active Voice

The style of active voice is

either

1. Subject-
2. Verb-
3. Object

or

1. Subject-
2. Verb

Passive Voice

The style of passive voice is either

1. Object
2. Verb
3. Subject

or

1. Object
2. Verb

Examples - Active voice versus Passive voice

Example 1:

We designed the cigar advertisement to appeal especially to the adolescent population.

vs.

Cigar advertisements were designed to appeal especially to the adolescent population.

Example 2:

Reducing Ca^{++} from the endoplasmic reticulum of the cell activates Ca^{++} channels.

vs.

The activation of Ca^{++} channels is induced by the reduction of endoplasmic reticulum Ca^{++} stores

3.3 Use Active Voice

While writing a medical research article, try writing an active voice. Be direct while writing the phrases.

1. The active voice is more lively and understandable.
2. It is a myth that avoiding first-person pronouns improves the objectivity of the paper.

3. You conducted the experiments and analyzed the findings. To suggest otherwise is deceptive.
4. The experiments and the subsequent analysis did not happen by chance! (For example, "the data were interpreted to demonstrate").
5. By agreeing to be an author for the scientific paper, you accept responsibility for its content. As a result, by using "we" or "I," you should claim responsibility for the text's assertions.

Is It Correct To Use "We" And "I"?

Yes. It's perfectly fine.

3.4 When Is It Appropriate to Use Passive Voice?

We can write the phrases in passive voice in the methods section. In the methods section,

- What was done matters more than who did it!
- Rather than reading the methods section as prose, readers tend to skim it for keywords.
- Avoiding the use of "we" and "I" in every sentence may take more effort than it is worth.

3.5 Handling Verbs

There are three rules to be followed while handling verbs in a sentence.
These rules are:

A. Use powerful verbs.
B. Avoid converting verbs to nouns.
C. Avoid burying the main verb.

A. Using strong verbs:

Verbs make sentences go! Pick the right verb!

Example:

In 2021, the WHO reports that more than sixty percent of diabetes patients in the world are found in developing countries, and estimates that the number of diabetics in these countries will double in the next 25 years.

In 2021, the WHO **estimates** that more than sixty percent of diabetes patients in the world are found in developing countries, and **projects** that the number of diabetics in these countries will double in the next 25 years.

B. Avoid turning verbs into nouns:

Avoid nominalization in writing wherever possible. Use verbs instead.

Table 3 Verbs and their noun counterparts

Verbs	Nouns
Provide a review of	Review
Has seen an expansion in	Has expanded
Obtain estimates of	Estimate
Give a description of	Describe
Shows a peak	Peaks
Offer confirmation of	Confirm
Take an assessment of	Assess

Example 1:

During DNA damage, recognition of H3K4me3 by ING2 results in recruitment of Sin3/HDAC and repression of cell proliferation genes.

(Ref: Miller JL, Grant PA. The role of DNA methylation and histone modifications in transcriptional regulation in humans. Subcell Biochem. 2013;61:289-317.)

Rewrite:

During DNA damage, H3K4me3 recruits ING2 and Sin3/HDAC, **which together repress cell** proliferation genes.

(Specify who does what to whom!)

C. Don't bury the primary verb:

Keep the subject and the main verb (predicate) close together at the start of the sentence. The verb is eagerly awaited by the readers!

Example 1:

The case of the buried predicate...

One study of 930 adults with multiple sclerosis (MS) receiving care in one of two managed care settings or in a fee-for-service setting found that only two-thirds of those needing to contact a neurologist for an MS-related problem in the prior 6 months had done so.

(Ref: Somerset M, Campbell R, Sharp DJ, Peters TJ. What do people with MS want and expect from health-care services? Health Expect. 2001 Mar;4(1):29-37.)

Possible rewrite:

One study found that, of 930 adults with multiple sclerosis (MS) who were receiving care in one of two managed care settings or in a fee-for-service setting, only two-thirds of those needing to contact a neurologist for an MS-related problem in the prior six months had done so.

3.6 Eliminate "to be" Verbs

Try eliminating "to be" verbs in writing where ever possible. The problems with to be verbs are:

1. They exaggerate their claim to permanence.
2. The "to be" verbs assert absolute truth and exclude all other points of view.
3. The verbs for "to be" are general and lack specificity.
4. The verbs that begin with "to be" are ambiguous.
5. The "to be" verbs frequently mislead the reader as to the subject of the sentence.

"To be" verbs	Replace with
Be	May be
Am	Will be
Been	Would be
Is	Shall be
Are	Should be
Was	Might be
Were	Could be
	Has been
	Must be

2.7 Watch Your Grammar

1. Data is plural, Datum is singular. For instance, 'Data are similar to urban population' NOT 'Data is similar to urban population'.

Examples:

The data are crucial.
The data support the conclusion.
These data express an unusual pattern.

2. Affect versus effect

Affect is a verb that means "to influence".

- The therapy affected her.
- Affect, which is a noun, denotes feeling or emotion expressed through words or body language, as in "The soldiers seen on television had been carefully chosen for their lack of emotion".

Effect is the noun form of this particular influence.

- The counseling had an effect on her.
- The verb "effect" means to bring about or cause a change, as in "to effect a change".

Examples:

1. The prescribed medication had an effect on the patients' symptoms.
2. How does the drug frequency affect metabolism in the liver?

3. Compared to versus compared with

Compare to = To highlight any similarities between two or more entities.

Compare with = To draw attention to differences between similar entities.

1. Shall I compare postpartum blues of normal women to hypothyroid women?
2. Brain tumors are uncommon in comparison to more common cancers, such as oral, lung and breast cancer.

4. That versus which

"That" is the restrictive pronoun that usually defines. "Which" is the nonrestrictive pronoun that is non-defining.

What's the difference between the following two sentences? Which one to use?

- The vial that contained her blood sample was lost.
- The vial, which contained her blood sample, was lost.

Consider the following: Is your clause essential or non-essential?

THAT: It is impossible to remove the essential clause without changing the meaning of the sentence.

WHICH: The non-essential clause can be removed without changing the basic meaning of the phrase (and must be set off by commas).

Example 1:

Other disorders **which** have been found to co-occur with diabetes include kidney disease and retinal problems.

Replace "which" with "that":

Other disorders **that** have been found to co-occur with diabetes include kidney disease and retinal problems.

Example 2:

Myocardial infarction incidence data are obtained from sources, **which** use the ICD.

Myocardial infarction incidence data are obtained from sources **that** use the ICD.

3.8 Assignments

Assignment 1:

Rewrite the sentences:

1. A recommendation was made by the ethics committee that the study be stopped.
2. Major differences in the blood sugar of the two study participants were found.
3. It was concluded by the editorial members that the data had been falsified by the authors.

Answers:

1. The ethics committee recommended that the study be stopped d.

2. We observed major differences in the blood sugar of the two study participants.
3. The editorial members concluded that the authors falsified their data.

Assignment 2:

Identify the issues and rewrite the sentences:

1. Review of each center's progress in recruitment is important to ensure that the cost involved in maintaining each center's participation is worthwhile.
2. It should be emphasized that these proportions generally are not the result of significant increases in moderate and severe injuries, but in many instances reflect mildly injured persons not being seen at a hospital.

Answers:

1. We should review each center's recruitment progress to make sure its continued participation is cost-effective.

Explanation:

- Inappropriate location of the verb
- Watch out for vague descriptors, such as "important" and "worthwhile"
- Clunky phrase
- "To be" is a weak verb

2. Shifting proportions in injury severity may reflect stricter hospital admission criteria rather than true increases in moderate and severe injuries.

Explanation:

- The phrase has an emphasis on deadweight
- More informative adjective than a pronoun - Why are these proportions important?
- Dead weight - generally. Consider the following: What does the sentence lose by not including this qualifier? Not using positives.

4

THE ART OF WRITING - PUNCTUATIONS IN THE RIGHT PLACES

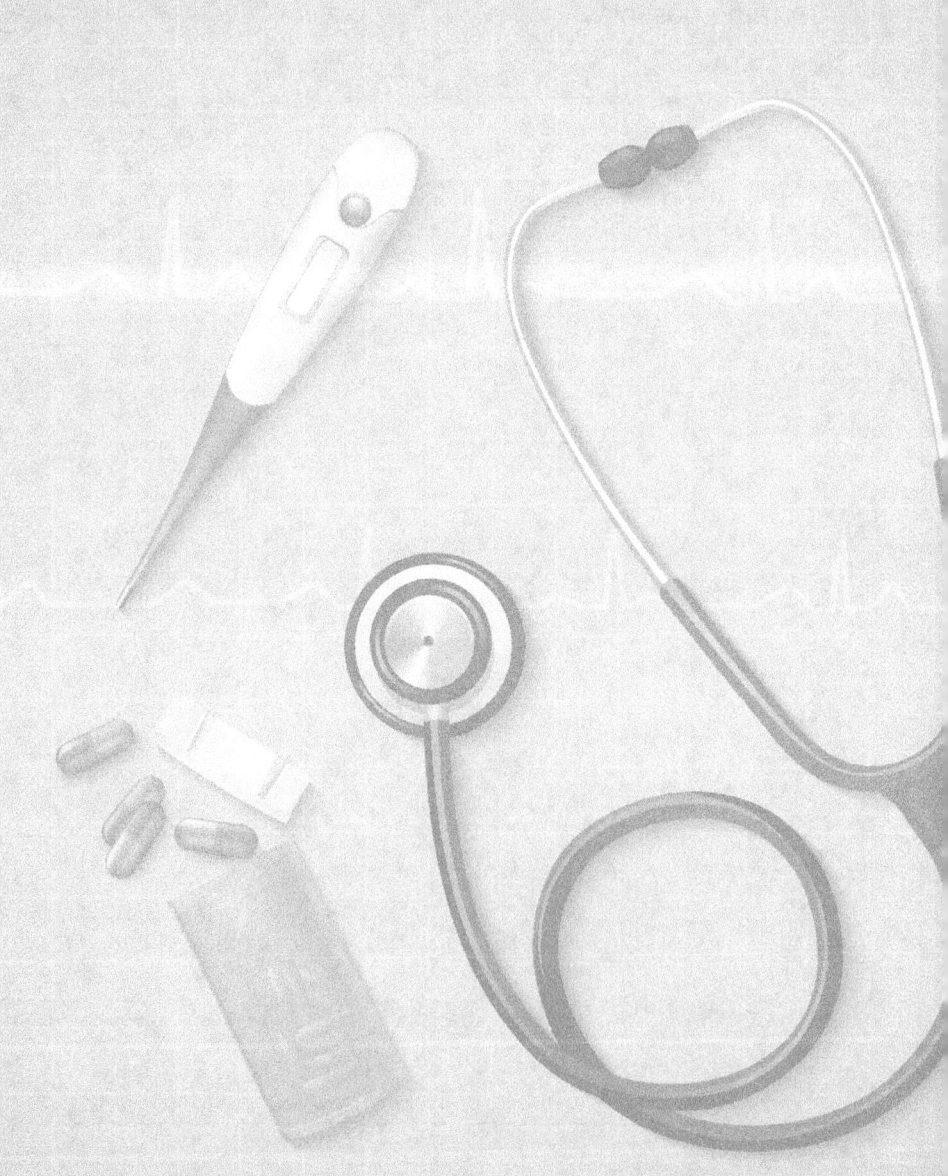

4.1 Introduction to Punctuations

Punctuation adds silent intonation to our writing. We use a comma, a period, an exclamation point, or a question mark to pause, stop, emphasize, or question, respectively. Correct punctuation improves the clarity and precision of writing by allowing the writer to stop, pause, or emphasize specific parts of the sentence.

You can't write if you don't use punctuation. You could, but your writing would be meaningless to your reader. Punctuation is as important as word choice, syntax, and structure in your writing. When any of these elements is missing, the result is a word salad rather than a coherent piece of writing.

Most salads are delicious, but word salad is not one of them. By becoming a punctuation expert, you can avoid serving up jumbled words. Use punctuations to vary sentence structure. Commonly used punctuations are dash, colon, semicolon, and parentheses.

Order of punctuations with increasing power to separate:

Period
Semicolon
Parentheses
Dash
Colon
Comma

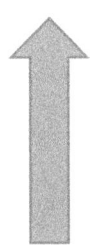

Order of punctuations with increasing formality:

Others (Comma, Colon, Semicolon, Period)
Parentheses
Dash

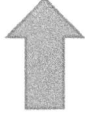

4.2 Colon

Colon is the most prevalent punctuation mark in sentences. When the second clause explains or illustrates the first, a colon is used to separate the two clauses.

Example 1:

Original:

Many different types of cells and tissues develop some degree of directionality. Certain events take place at either end of the cell or tissue. Cell polarity is a biological phenomenon.

Using a colon: Many cells and tissues develop a type of directionality known as cell polarity: certain events occur at one end of the cell or tissue.

What not to do with a colon!

Example:

In the WHO project, we have a psychologist, clinicians, a nutritionist, statisticians, and dietitians: robust manpower.

Rewrite:

In the WHO project, we have robust manpower: a psychologist, clinicians, a nutritionist, statisticians, and dietitians.

4.3 Semicolon

Two independent clauses are separated by a semicolon. A clause is a grammatical organization element that comes after a sentence and always has a subject and predicate. The first word after the semicolon, like the colon, should not be capitalized unless it is typically capitalized. In lists with internal punctuation, semicolons are also used to separate items.

Example 1:

Kennedy could be a cold and vain man, and he led a life of privilege. But he knew something about the world; he also cared about it.

Example 2:

It was the best of times; it was the worst of times.

4.4 Parenthesis

Parenthesis marks are used in pairs; the plural is "parentheses". This is how parentheses look: ( ). When you use parentheses to separate material in a sentence, you say it's "in parenthesis". Put something in parentheses if it's a remark, an afterthought, or extra information, which might be interesting but isn't necessary for the subject.

Use parentheses to insert an afterthought or explanation (a word, phrase, or sentence) into a grammatically complete passage.

- If the material within the parentheses is removed, the main point of the sentence should not change.
- Parentheses allow the reader to skip ahead in the text.

Example 1:

This is concerning because, while there are plausible biological explanations for the link between red meat and cancer and heart disease, it appears unlikely that eating too much red meat could directly cause accidents and injuries. (Unless, as one of the researchers observed, red meat eaters swerve to avoid goats!)

4.5 Dash

Use a dash to add emphasis or to insert an abrupt definition or description almost anywhere in the sentence. Just don't overdo it, or it will lose its potency.

"A dash is a mark of separation stronger than a comma, less formal than a colon, and more relaxed than parentheses."— Strunkand White

Example 1:

The newer drugs did more than preventing new fat accumulation. They also triggered the obese rabbits to lose bulk fat—more than half their body weight.

What effect would parentheses or commas have on the tone of these sentences?

- Instead of commas...
  (clumsy and lengthy...)

The newer drugs did more than just keep new fat from accumulating. They also caused obese rabbit to lose significant fat, more than half their body weight.

- Instead, use parentheses...
  (buries the information)

The newer drugs did more than just keep new fat from accumulating. They also caused obese rabbit to lose a significant amount of fat (more than half their body weight).

4.5 Parallelism

Grammar defines parallelism as two or more phrases or clauses in a sentence that have the same grammatical structure. Lists of ideas (including numbered lists of ideas) should be written parallel to one another. Ideas connected by "and", "or", or "but" should be written in parallel form.

Example 1:

Not parallel:

If you want to be a successful doctor, you must study hard, think critically about the medical conditions, and you should be a good observer.

Parallel:

If you want to be a successful doctor you must study hard, observe well, and think critically about the medical conditions. (imperative, imperative, imperative)

Or

If you want to be a good doctor, you must be a good student, a good listener, and a critical thinker about medical literature. (noun, noun, noun)

4.6 Paragraphs

One paragraph = One concept

Give the punch line right away. The logical flow of ideas aids in graph flow.

If parallel sentence structures are required, use transition words. The first and last sentences will be remembered the most by your reader. Make the last sentence stand out by emphasizing it. The emphasis is at the very end!

Flow of ideas logically:

- Time-sequenced (avoid the Memento method!)
- Generalized messages followed by specific ones (key message first!)
- Logical reasoning (if a then b; a; therefore b)

4.7 Repetition

When you find yourself reaching for the thesaurus to avoid using the same word twice in the same sentence or even paragraph.

Consider the following:

1. Is the second occurrence of the word even required?
2. If the word is required, is a synonym really preferable to simply repeating the word?

- It is acceptable to repeat words. Resist the urge to shorten words simply because they appear frequently! (Recall that miR stands for microRNA rather than microRNA).
- Only use standard acronyms/initialisms (e.g., RNA). They are not made up!
- If you must use acronyms, define them in the abstract, each table/figure, and the text separately. If you're writing

a long paper, redefine it now and then (because most readers don't read from beginning to end).

ASSIGNMENT:

Use punctuations wherever applicable

1. Evidence-based medicine teaches clinicians the practical application of clinical epidemiology, as needed to address specific problems of specific patients. It guides clinicians on how to find the best evidence relevant to a specific problem, how to assess the quality of that evidence, and perhaps most difficult, how to decide if the evidence applies to a specific patient.

2. Finally, the lessons of clinical epidemiology are not meant to be limited to academic physician-epidemiologists, who sometimes have more interest in analyzing data than caring for patients. Clinical epidemiology holds the promise of providing clinicians with the tools necessary to improve the outcomes of their patients.

(Ref: Masic I, Miokovic M, Muhamedagic B. Evidence based medicine - new approaches and challenges. Acta Inform Med. 2008;16(4):219-25)

Answers:

1. Evidence-based medicine teaches clinicians the practical application of clinical epidemiology: how to find the best evidence relevant to a specific problem, how to assess the quality of that evidence, and how to decide if the evidence applies to a specific patient.

Or

Evidence-based medicine teaches clinicians how to find the best evidence relevant to a specific problem, how to assess the quality of that evidence, and how to decide if the evidence applies to a specific patient.

2. Finally, clinical epidemiology is not limited to academic physician-epidemiologist - who are sometimes more interested in analyzing data than caring for patients - but provides clinicians with the tools to improve their patients' outcomes.

Explanation:

- No transition
- A long descriptive clause that could be set off by a dash

PARAGRAPH PRACTICE

Example:

Previous research has consistently found an increased risk of subsequent drug use associated with conduct problems and antisocial behavior in childhood, and a general survey of young adults found an association between drug dependence and conduct problems. Furthermore, long-term relationships between aggressive, unconventional, and impulsive behaviors and drug use involvement, in general, have been discovered. However, there may be multiple pathways between early childhood misbehavior and drug use. Psychiatric symptoms and cognitive disabilities can manifest as aggressive behaviors, and drug use can be a reaction to impulsive tendencies, which frequently co-occur with aggression or misbehavior. Distress and a failure to adopt responsible traditional roles and behaviors may be important mediators in the link between childhood misbehavior and late drug dependence.

Answer:

Possible rewrite:

Previous research has linked early childhood behavioral issues to later drug use. According to studies, young adults and adult drug users are more aggressive, unconventional, and impulsive than their peers. Several pathways may account for our findings: aggressive children may have underlying psychiatric disorders or cognitive disabilities that increase their risk of drug use; misbehavior tends to co-occur with impulsivity, which increases the risk of drug use; and childhood misbehavior may lead to long-term problems, such as persistent distress or a failure to ever adopt conventional roles or behaviors, which may lead to drug dependence.

5

WRITING STRATEGY

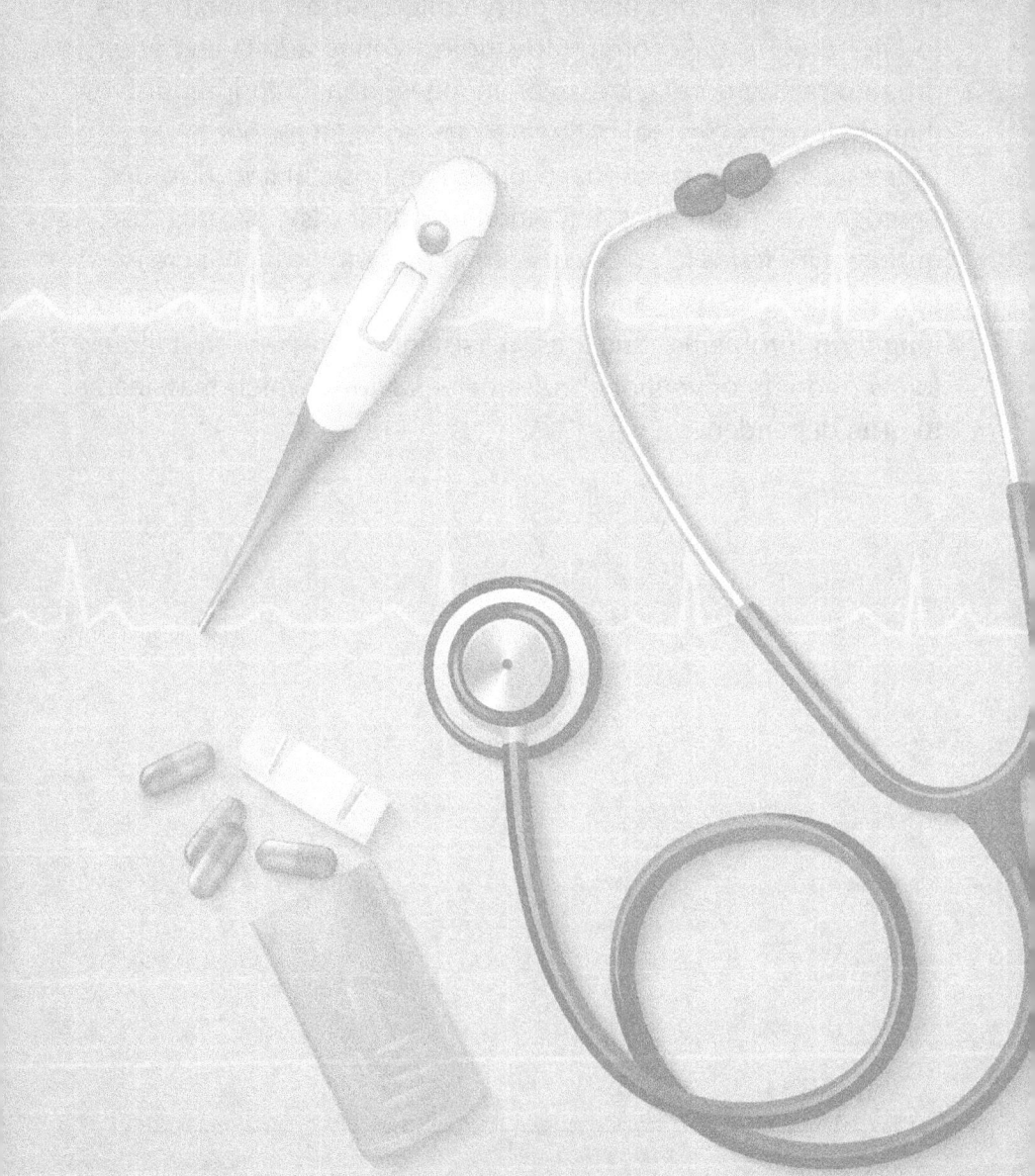

Much progress has been made in the field of medical writing. Editors reject poorly prepared manuscripts and work to improve those that are accepted. Referees provide detailed criticism of the content of papers submitted, allowing a journal to maintain its high standards despite the volume of work submitted to it. However, many authors have difficulty placing a piece of writing that has taken a long time and effort to prepare and may contain important work. A medical author should strive to be all of the following: original, honest, innovative, well-organized, cautious, clear, modest, fair-minded, forthright, persistent, rigorous, and realistic. These characteristics are critical. To accomplish this, the style and format must be appropriate.

5.1 Steps in the Writing Process

1. Prewriting
- Assemble, synthesize, and organize data
- Make a list of take-home messages;
- Get ideas out of your head and away from the computer.
- Make a road map or outline.

2. Writing the first draft

- Organizing your facts and ideas into an organized sentence

3. Revision

- Read your work aloud
- Remove clutter
- Perform a verb check
- Gather feedback from others

How much time do you think you can allocate to each of the following steps proportionally?

1. Prewriting
2. Writing
3. Revision

Roughly, the time allocation is as follows: rewriting - 70%, writing the first draft - 10%, and revision - 20%.

5.2 The Pre-writing Step

Tips for pre-writing:

5.2.1 First, get organized!

- Do not attempt to write and gather information at the same time!
- Collect and organize all required information before writing the first draft.

5.2.2 Organizing your thoughts:

- Do you have a system in place to keep track of things?
- If you don't have one, make one for yourself!
- Spend less time writing and more time organizing. Simply put, it's less painful!

5.2.3 Make a road map for yourself:

- Before starting to write the first draft, make a rough road map/outline with key information and citations from the scientific literature.
- Consider your ideas in paragraphs and sections...

5.2.4 Do a Brainstorm while you are away from the computer:

- While you're on the go, write!
- While doing workouts (turn off your airpod)
- When you're alone in the car (turn off the radio!)
- While standing in the queue (Put your magazine down!)
- Make a filing system for your papers.
- Come up with catchy lines

5.2.5 Compositional structure:

- Relatively similar paragraphs must be grouped.
- Don't constantly "bait and switch" your reader.
- Use the following formula when debating a point of contention: All counter-arguments, rebuttals, and arguments (all)

5.3 The Writing Step

Initial tips for writing the first draft:

- Avoid being a perfectionist!
- The goal of the first draft is to get the ideas down in full sentences and in the correct order. Pay greater attention to the logical organization than to sentence-level specifics.
- For most people, the first draft is the most difficult phase. Reduce the discomfort by completing the first draft swiftly and efficiently!

Example:

First draft:

In this era of 'all work and no play', in a desire to get ahead in their work-place, people are often undertaking new projects at the expense of good sleep giving rise to a 24-hour society with increasing prevalence of unusual work hours.

(Ref: Nirupama AY, Vinoth Gnana Chellaiyan D, Ravivarman G. Is Adequate Sleep Becoming Outlandish Among Healthcare Professionals? - A Review on Its Toll on Their Health. Natl J Community Med 2021;12(12):444-448.)

Revised version:

In this era of 'all work and no play,' people are frequently undertaking new projects at the expense of adequate sleep, resulting in a 24-hour society with an increasing prevalence of unusual work hours.

5.3 Revision

Tips on revision:

- Read your work aloud
- Check for verbs
- Remove clutter
- Review your organization
- Get comments from others
- Hire an editor

5.3.1 Read your writing out loud

The brain processes the spoken word differently than the written word!

5.3.2 Do a verb check

In each sentence, highlight the main verb. Look out for:

(1) Verbs that lack luster (e.g., There are many first-year medical students who struggle with histology.)

(2) Verbs that are inactive (e.g., The reaction was noted by her.)

5.3.3 Cut clutter

Don't be afraid to cut!

Watch out for:

- Deadweight words and phrases (it should be emphasized that)
- Empty words and phrases (basic tenets of, important)
- Long words or phrases that could be short (muscular and cardiorespiratory performance)
- Unnecessary jargon and acronyms
- Repetitive words or phrases (teaches clinicians/guides clinicians)
- Adverbs (very, really, quite, basically)

5.3.4 Conduct an organizational audit

Each paragraph should be labeled in the margins of your paper with a phrase or sentence that summarizes the main point. Then, rearrange paragraphs to improve logical flow and group similar ideas together.

5.3.5 Get feedback from others

- Request that your manuscript be read by someone outside of your department.
- Request that someone not related to your department read your manuscript.

- o They should be able to understand the following even if they have no technical background: the key findings
- o Messages to take home
- o The importance of your work
- Request that they point out any sentences or paragraphs that are particularly difficult to read!

5.3.6 Get help

- Hire a professional editor to proofread your work!
- The checklist for the final draught
  - ➢ Examine for consistency.
  - ➢ Examine for numerical consistency.
  - ➢ Examine your references.

Check for consistency

"We followed participants for a minimum of 2 years." (Methods section)
"The average follow-up time was 1.5 years." (Results section)

Check for numerical consistency

Do the total numbers in the abstract match the total numbers in your text/tables/figures?

- Do the numbers of tables/figures in the text match?
- Do the numbers in each table/figure correspond to the numbers in other tables/figures?

Check your references

- Do you have "references to nowhere"?

- A reference does not provide the indicated information/ fact. Authors misinterpreted or exaggerated the findings from the original source.
- Reference cites a secondary source rather than a primary source. (Citation propagation!)
- The authors misnumbered the references.

> **Nuggets**
>
> - Always cite/go back to primary sources!
>
> - Assume that other authors have made errors in citing sources!

6

PLAGIARISM

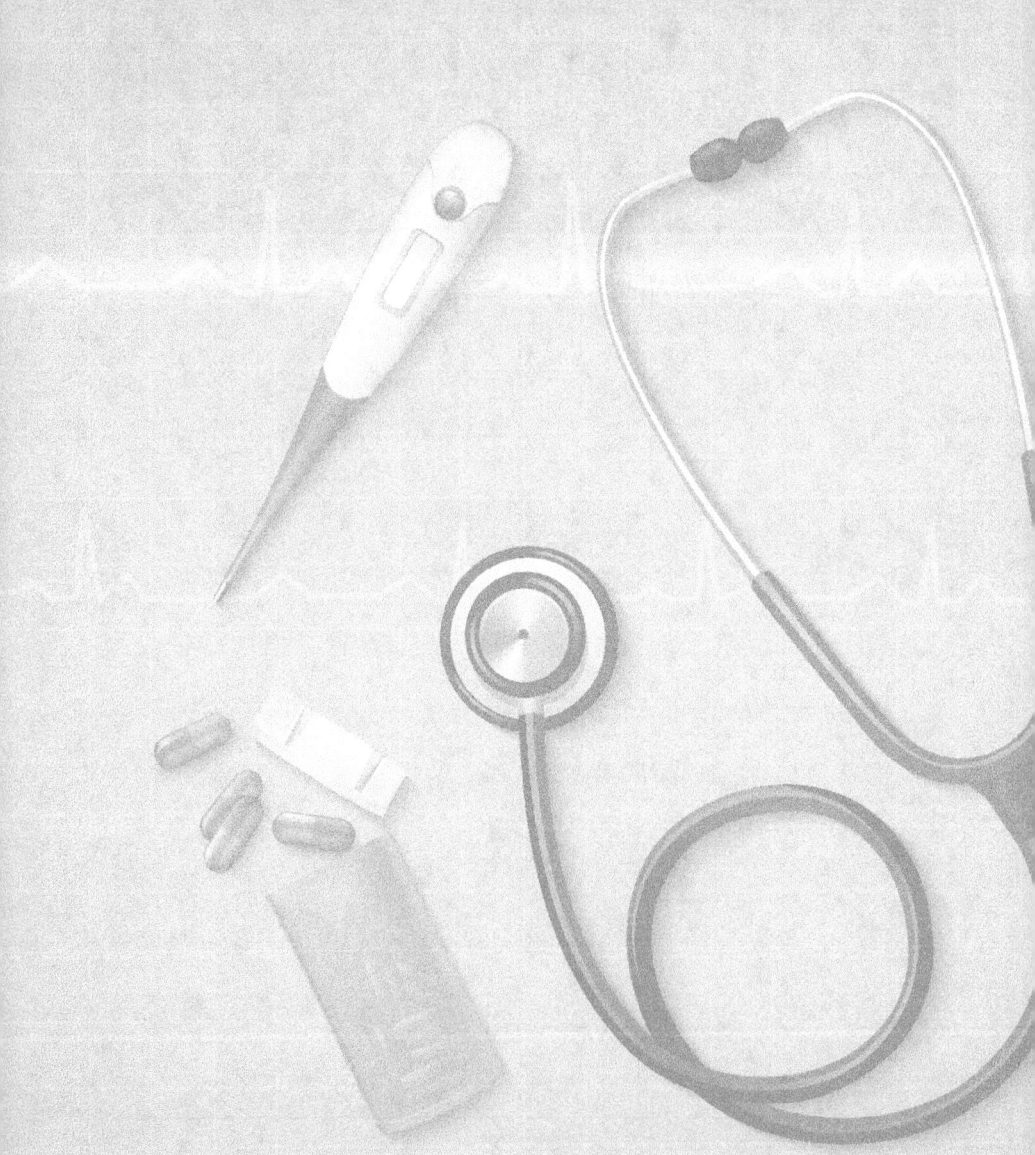

The essence of good medical writing, or any type of scientific writing is a clear, succinct, precise, and honest explanation of the scientific idea.

6.1 What is plagiarism?

Plagiarism is defined as misrepresenting someone else's work or idea as one's own without properly crediting the source. Plagiarism is defined as misrepresenting someone else's work or idea as one's own without properly crediting the source. Plagiarism is probably the most well-known unethical practice in medical writing. Plagiarism can manifest itself in a variety of ways, some of which are subtle and do not constitute scientific misconduct. Others may constitute misappropriation, and thus scientific misconduct, with ethical and legal consequences. It refers to misrepresenting someone else's writing as your own.

This includes:

- Taking sentences or even phrases from another source and pasting them;
- Slightly rewriting or rearrangement of others' words; and
- Borrowing material from websites such as Wikipedia.

6.2 Types of Plagiarism

Plagiarism can be classified into several types. They are as follows:

1. **Plagiarism of ideas**
   Even if an author does not duplicate any words or phrases from the original piece, plagiarism may occur if he just

utilizes the same concept, idea, or creation and presents it as his own without proper acknowledgment. This type of plagiarism is difficult to detect, but it is a significant offense once discovered.

It is a regular occurrence among postgraduate students who get ideas for their thesis papers by looking at previous research publications. Faculty members at some institutions are often unconcerned about such tactics and students have been instructed by their guides to pick up a thesis that is more than 5 years old and rewrite it as a new study.

During seminar and conference presentations, plagiarized ideas are also prevalent. Other instances of plagiarism of ideas include reviewers hijacking the ideas of students, authors, or principal investigators.

2. **Plagiarism of text**
    Text plagiarism is also known as "word-for-word" plagiarism.

    "...copying a chunk of content from another source without providing acknowledgment to its creator and without enclosing the borrowed text in quote marks."

    Previously, plagiarizing text from an article required a lot of effort. To be able to duplicate relevant concepts and material, one had to go to libraries, read a lot of literature, and go through multiple textbooks. Even the availability of such resources was limited. Plagiarism is very simple thanks to technological advancements. The practice appears to have grown in popularity as a result of widespread internet access, simply because the material is readily available online and may be copied. "Cut-copy-paste" appears to be a global phenomenon.

3. **Self-plagiarism**

   The author may borrow heavily from his or her own previous work at times. The reader expects to read original articles in scientific journals, and any form of self-plagiarism violates those expectations.

   Reusing your own writing or data, such as:
   - Text from previously published papers that have been copied or only slightly rewritten.
   - Adding new data to previously published data and displaying them as new results
   - Submitting data that is identical to or overlapping that provided in multiple journals.

4. **Mosaic plagiarism**

   Mosaic plagiarism is defined as "... borrowing ideas and opinions from an original source, as well as a few verbatim words or phrases without crediting the original author." The plagiarist, in this case, mingles his or her own ideas and opinions with those of the original author, resulting in a muddled, plagiarized mass.

   When the original author is not acknowledged and the reference is not properly cited, the interlacing is considered plagiarism.

6.3 How to Avoid Plagiarism?

Tips for writing about other people's ideas/work:

- You must comprehend the material thoroughly enough to express it in your own words!
- Use your memory to work.

- Come to your own conclusions.
- Do not simply re-arrange the original author's words or mimic the original author's sentence structure.

6.4 Software that detect plagiarism

In recent days, it is easy to detect plagiarism with the help of software. Some are free and some come with a price.

Given below is a list of some software that detect plagiarism:

1. Plagiarism Checker X
2. Grammarly
3. Copyscape
4. Ginger
5. Plagscan
6. Plagiarisma
7. Duplichecker
8. Turnitin Plagiarism Checker
9. Urkund Plagiarism Checker
10. iThenticate Plagiarism Detection Software
11. CopyLeaks Plagiarism Detector
12. Quetext
13. PaperRater
14. Plagium
15. Plagly

Example 1:

Original paper (2004): "Although earlier registry-based analyses of second neoplasms after breast cancer (BC) did not detect an increased risk of cutaneous melanoma (CM),[1][2] several more recent registry-based[3][4] and hospital-based[5] studies have documented a statistically significant increased risk of CM after BC with standardized incidence ratios (SIRs) ranging from 1.4 to 2.7."

Second paper (2009): "Recent registry-based [1,2] and hospital-based [3,4] studies have documented a statistically significant increased risk of CM after BC with standardized incidence ratios (SIRs) ranging from 1.4 to 2.7."

Plagiarism: References 1, 2, 3, and 4 are identical

Other considerations when writing an article

6.5 Ghostwriting, Gift, and Guest Authorship

Ghost authors:
Writers-for-hire who draft manuscripts (usually for companies), but are not listed as authors.

Gift authorship:
The practice of giving gift authorship is widespread in many institutions and has grown in popularity in recent years. Gift authorship is defined as co-authorship given to someone who did not make a significant contribution to the study. There are several reasons why someone might write a gift. Junior researchers are frequently pressed to accept or assign authorship to senior colleagues who wield significant power over their future careers. Furthermore, junior researchers may believe that adding more senior colleagues as authors will increase their chances of publication. Senior investigators may grant gift authorship to encourage collaboration and maintain good working relationships, or as remuneration for favors. Gift

authorship, regardless of the reason, is an unacceptable practice in academic publications.

Guest or "honorary" authors:
Academic researchers who are minimally involved in a paper, but "lend" their name as an author (often first author!) to bolster the paper's credibility.

6.6 Conflicts of Interest/Disclosure

Any financial or personal relationship that might influence (bias) an author's, reviewer's, or editor's judgments. (International Committee of Medical Journal Editors)
Conflicts of interest:

- Should be disclosed (most biomedical journals require this),
- May influence an editor's (or reviewer's) decision to reject or accept a paper and
- Are often printed in a published paper.

7

REFERENCING

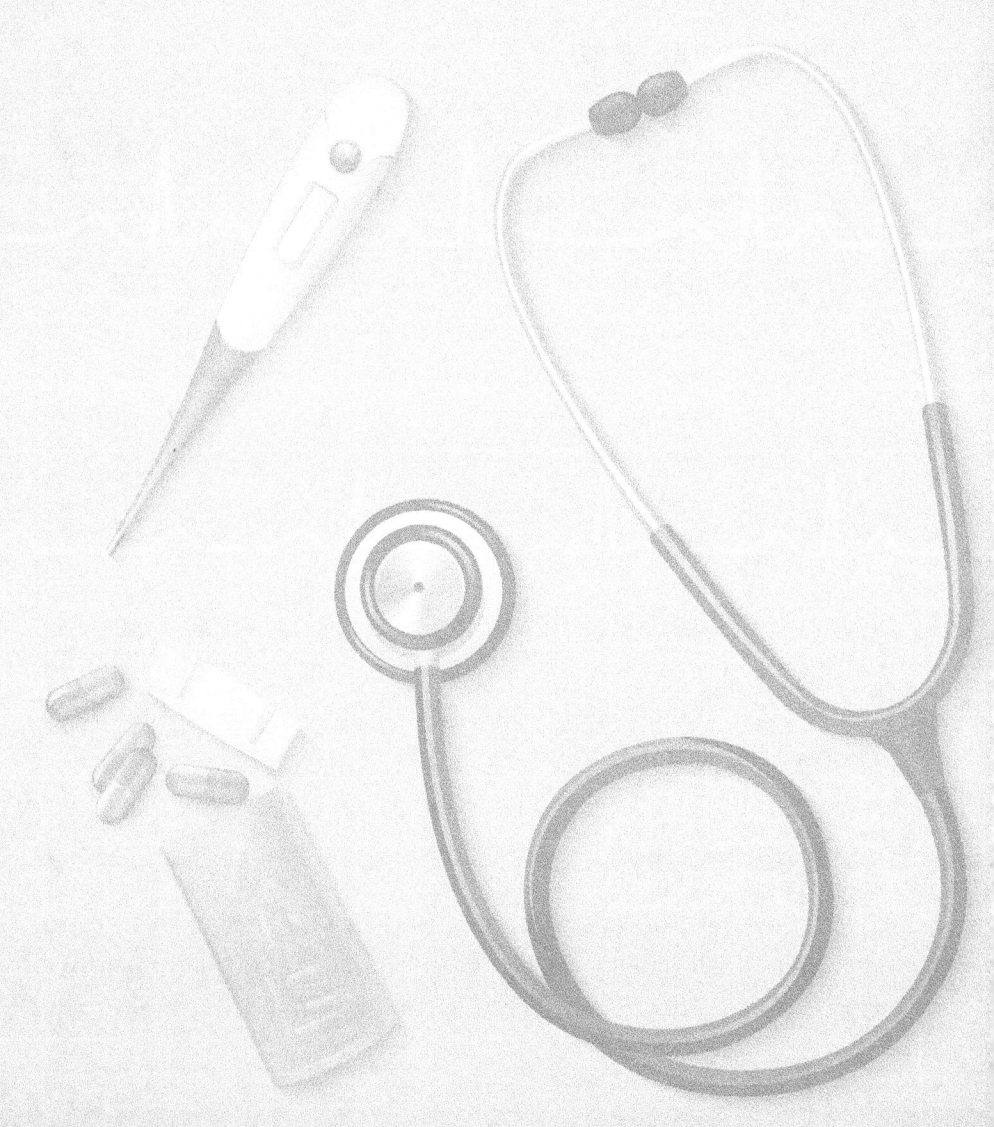

7.1 What is Referencing?

It's a technique for demonstrating to your audience that you've conducted an extensive and relevant literature search and reading. Similarly, referencing acknowledges that you borrowed ideas and written material from other authors and used them in your own work. This referencing style has two parts: citations and the reference list.

7.2 Need to Reference

1. Appropriate referencing is an important part of good academic practice because it demonstrates that your writing is founded on knowledge and informed by appropriate academic reading.
2. You will ensure that anyone who reads your work can find the sources you used to create it and credit you for your research efforts and quality.
3. You may be charged with plagiarism if you do not acknowledge the work or ideas of others...

7.3 Citation

You must acknowledge this in the text of your work when you use another person's work in your own, whether by referring to their ideas or including a direct quotation. A citation is a type of acknowledgment like this.

7.4 Bibliography

There may be products that you used in your research but did not cite. These can be listed in a 'bibliography' at the end of your project. These items should be organized alphabetically by author and formatted identically to the references in your bibliography. You won't need a reference list if you can cite every source you used.

If you want to show your reader any unused research you completed, include it in the bibliography. Each work in your bibliography does not need to be numbered.

7.5 How to Choose a Citation Style?

Sometimes, citation depends upon the academic discipline involved and as per journal requirements. There are five major styles of citation.

- APA (American Psychological Association) is used by Education, Psychology, and Sciences
- MLA(Modern Language Association) style is used by the humanities
- Chicago/Turbian style is generally used by Business, History, and Fine Arts
- Harvard style is a brief citation to a source and is given in parentheses within the text of an article
- Vancouver is most commonly used in medical journals

7.6 Software for Writing References

There are several software available for referencing any content.

1. Zotero
2. EndNote
3. Flowcite
4. RefWork
5. Mendeley
6. Citationsy

7.7 Vancouver Style from Various Sources

1. Journal articles (printed)

Required items:

- Author names
- Initials
- Title
- Name of the Journal
- Year
- Volume
- Issue
- Page numbers

If a reference has up to six authors, list all of them in your reference list; if there are more than six, list the top six authors followed by the term "et al.".

Examples:

1) Simon ST, Kini V, Levy AE, Ho PM. Medication adherence in cardiovascular medicine. BMJ. 2021 Aug 11;374:n1493. pmid:34380627.

2) Bauer AM, Parker MM, Schillinger D, Katon W, Adler N, Adams AS, et al. Associations between antidepressant adherence and shared decision-making, patient-provider trust, and communication among adults with diabetes: diabetes study of Northern California (DISTANCE). J Gen Intern Med. 2014 Aug;29(8):1139–1147.

2. Journal articles (electronic)

Required items:

- Author names
- Title
- Name of the Journal
- Year
- Volume
- Issue
- Page numbers
- Cited date
- Website where the content is available

Examples:

1) Zylka MJ, Simon JM, Philpot BD. Gene length matters in neurons. Neuron [Internet]. 2015 [cited 2021 Jul 22];86(2):353-5. Available from: Medline (For library subscribed database)
2) Montagner AF, Carvalho MPM, Susin AH. Microshear bonding effectiveness of different regions. Indian J Dent Res [Internet]. 2015 [cited 2021 Jun 29];26(2):131-135. Available from: http://www.ijdr.in/article.asp?issn= 09709290;year=2015;volume=26;issue=2;spage= 131;epage=135;aulast=Montagner (from the internet)

3. Printed book

Required items:

- Number
- Author/Editor
- Title **of the book**

- Sub-title
- Edition
- Place of the publication
- Year

Examples:

1) Strom BL, Kimmel SE. Textbook of Pharmacoepidemiology. John Wiley. 2013.
2) Jenkins PF. Making sense of the chest x-ray: a hands-on guide. New York: Oxford University Press; 2005. 194 p.

4. E-book

Required items:

- Author(s)
- Title of book
- [Internet]
- Edition
- Place of publication
- Year
- [cited in year month date format]
- [Available from: web link]

Example:

Warrell DA, Cox TM, Firth JD, editors. Oxford textbook of medicine [Internet]. Oxford: Oxford University Press; 2015 [cited 2021 Jul 14]. Available from: http://oxfordmedicine.com/view/10.1093/med/9780199204854.001.1/med-9780199204854

5. Website

Required items:

- Author/Organization
- Title of the study
- Internet
- Place of the publication
- Publisher name
- Updated year month date; cited year month date
- Available from: (web link)

Example:

World Health Organization. Drinking water [Internet]. Switzerland: World health Organization; 2015 Jun [cited 2022 Jan 20]. Available from: http://www.who.int/mediacentre/factsheets/fs391/en/

6. Newspaper article

Required items:

- Author (If author details are not available, use the title in italics)
- Title of article
- Title of newspaper
- Year-month-date
- Page reference

Example:

Tynan T. Medical improvements lower homicide rate: study sees drop in assault rate. The Washington Post. 2002 Aug 12;Sect. A:2 (col. 4).

7. Conference proceedings

Required items:

- Author's names with initials
- Title of paper
- Complete title of the conference in upper case
- Year, month, date of the conference
- Location
- Add details of place and publisher (if published)

Example:

Castillo RR, Abarquez RF, Aquino AV, Sy RG, Gomez LA, Divinagracia RA, et al. editors. 10th Asia Pacific congress of hypertension – APCH 2014; 2014 Feb 12-15; Cebu City (Philippines). Florence (Italy): Monduzzi Editore, International Proceedings Division; c2014.

8. Printed Government reports

Required items:

- Organization name
- Title of the report
- Paper number
- Place of publication
- Publisher details
- Year of publication

Example:

Continuity of Care With Family Medicine Physicians: Why It Matters. Canadian Institute for Health Information (CIHI). Ottawa, ON. 2015.

9. Online government reports

Required items:

- Organization name
- Title of the report
- Paper number
- Internet
- Year of publication
- cited date
- Available from: URL (web link)

Example:

Department of Health. Equity and excellence: liberating the NHS, CM7881. [Internet]. 2010 [cited 2022 Jan 9]. Available from: https://www.dh.gov.uk/en/Publicationsandstatistics/ Publications/PublicationsPolicyAndGuidance/DH_117353

10. Reports from an organization - Print

Required items:

- Organization name
- Title of the report
- Paper number
- Place of publication
- Publisher name
- Year of publication

Example:

WHO. Strategy for malaria elimination in the Greater Mekong subregion (2015–2030). Geneva: World Health Organization, 2015

11. Reports from organization - Online

Required items:

- Organization name
- Title of the report
- Paper number
- Edition
- Internet in square brackets
- Year
- Cited date
- Available from: website link

Example:

General Medical Council. Good medical practice: working with doctors working for patients. Rev ed. [Internet]. 2014 [cited 2021 Nov 19]. Available from: https://www.gmc-uk.org/-/media/ documents/Good medical practice English 1215.pdf 51527435.pdf

12. Articles not in English

Required items:

- Authors names
- Title of study
- Language in square brackets
- Standard abbreviated title of journal
- Year, first three letters of the month, date
- Volume and issue number
- Page numbers (without p)

Example:

Miyazaki K, Murakami A, Imamura S, et al. A case of fundus albipunctatus with a retinol dehydrogenase 5 gene mutation in a child [in Japanese], Nippon Ganka Gakkat Zasshi. 2001; 105(8):530–534.

8

HOW TO WRITE A RESEARCH PROTOCOL

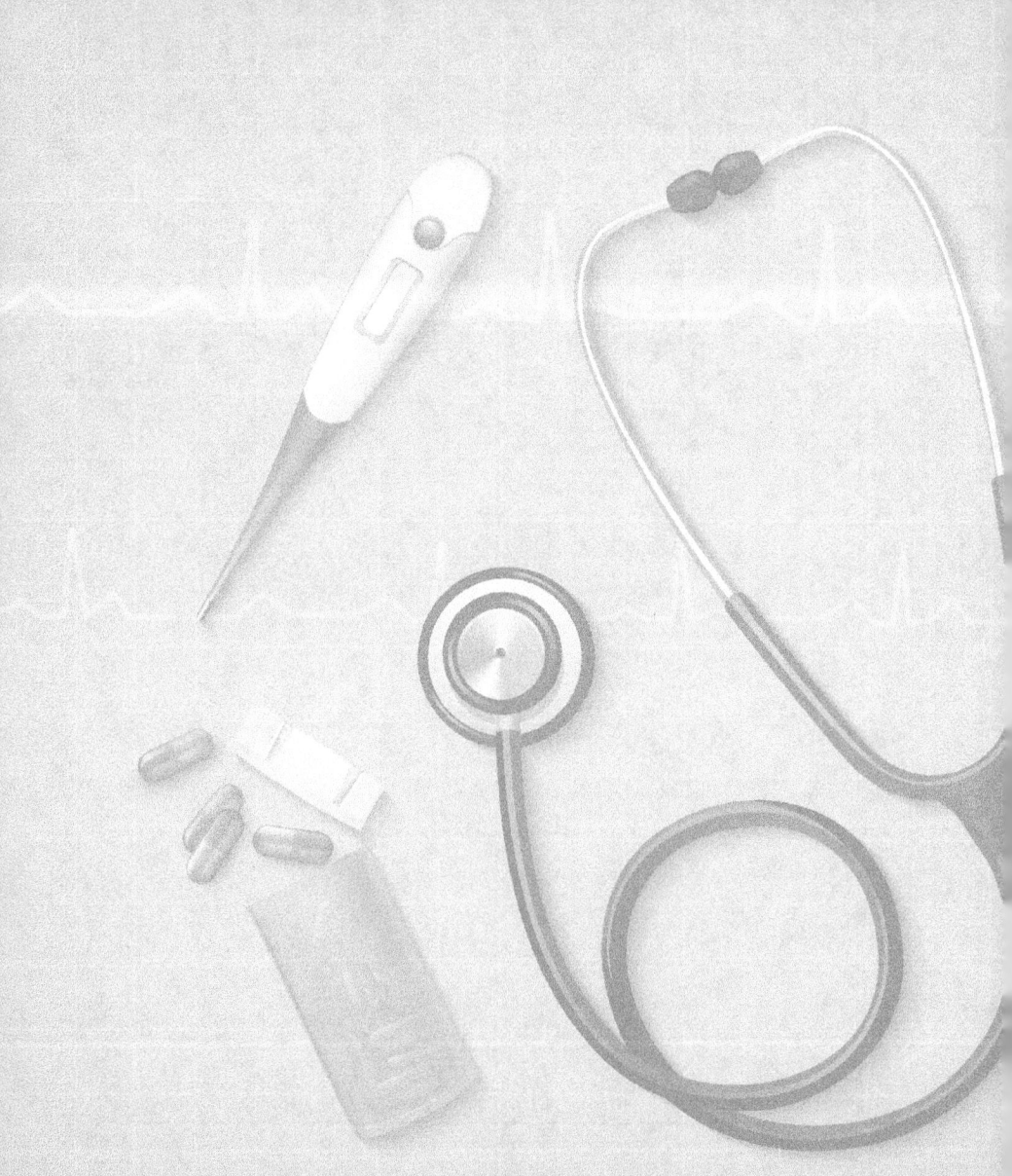

A proposal is a precise strategy or 'blueprint' for the proposed study, and once finalized, the research endeavor should run smoothly. The purpose of a research proposal is to describe the author's plan for the research they want to do. Part of this purpose, in some situations, is to gain money for the research. In certain cases, it's to get the author's supervisor or department to approve the research so they may proceed forward with it. A research proposal is sometimes requested as part of a graduate school application. The structure of research proposals is the same in all of these situations.

8.1 Steps of a Research Study

The steps in conducting a research study are as follows:

Choosing the research question

Developing the protocol

Pretesting and revising the protocol

Carrying out the study

Analyzing the findings

Drawing and disseminating the conclusion

8.2 Contents of a Protocol

A complete research proposal should have the following contents:

- ❑ Research question and hypothesis generation
- ❑ Title of the study
- ❑ Introduction
- ❑ Review of literature and lacunae
- ❑ Objectives
- ❑ Materials and methods
- ❑ Ethics considerations
- ❑ References
- ❑ Annexures

8.3 Research Question

A clear, well-thought-out proposal serves as the foundation for the research, making it the most significant step in the research process. Finding the research question for your study is the first step in preparing a proposal.

Ideas for new research could be started from:

- Professional experience
- Burning questions
- Literature
- Professional meetings
- Discussions

Any research study should fulfill FINER criteria.

- Feasible
- Interesting
- Novel

- Ethical
- Relevant

F stands for "feasible". Is it possible to answer the question? Do you have all of the materials you'll need to complete the research? Do you have enough subjects to choose from? Will you have sufficient time and funds? Do you have the necessary experience to conduct this research or can you work with someone who does?

I stands for "interesting". The research question must pique the investigator's attention, but it should also pique the interest of others.

N stands for "novel". Is this a new study or has it been done before? Does it contribute to the existing corpus of medical knowledge?

E stands for "ethical". Is it possible to conduct the study without endangering the participants? Will the study be approved by an IRB?

R stands for "relevant". Is it going to help medical science? Will the findings have an impact on clinical practice?

Question 1:

Does the following study fulfill FINER criteria?

Liraglutide Effect and Action in Diabetes: Evaluation of Cardiovascular Outcome Results

Answer:

1. Yes.

Explanation:
The goal of the trial was to assess the cardiovascular (CV) safety of liraglutide in patients with type 2 diabetes mellitus (T2DM) at high risk for CV events.

Contribution to the literature: The LEADER trial showed that liraglutide, a glucagon-like peptide-1 (GLP-1) agonist, was superior to placebo in improving glycemic control and reducing the risk of CV events in patients with T2DM and high CV risk.

Research Question and Hypothesis

After a research question is made, a research hypothesis needs to be made. Research hypothesis mentions the key elements of the study - the sample size, the study design, the predictor, and the outcome variables.

Example 1:

Research question:
Reading a book on research methodology is a boring task??

Hypothesis:
Reading a book on research methodology is a boring task compared with clinical work.

Framing a Research Question:
The research question should have the following elements on the basis of study designs:

- PO - Descriptive studies (cross-sectional)
- P.E.O. - (E-exposure) cohort, case-control
- P.I.C.O. - Clinical trials
- P.I.C.O.T. - Clinical trial, Meta-analysis

(POPULATION, INTERVENTION, CONTROL, OUTCOME, EXPOSURE, TIME FRAME)

Patient or Problem: Describe patients and their problems.

Intervention: Describe the main intervention, exposure, and test or prognostic factor under consideration.

Comparison: In the case of treatment, describe a comparative intervention. A comparison is not always needed

Outcome: Describe what you hope to achieve, measure, or affect.

Time: Describe the time frame for conducting the study.

Example 1: Descriptive study

Prevalence of electrocardiograph changes among Dengue fever patients attending the outpatient department of your hospital
PO:
Population - Patients with dengue fever
Outcome - ECG findings

Example 2: Case control study

Association Between Occupational Heat Stress and Kidney Disease Among Workers in the Thai Cohort Study
PEO:
Population - Thai workers
Exposure - Occupational heat stress
Outcome - Kidney disease

Example 3: Clinical trials

Effects of Nasal Calcitonin vs. Oral Gabapentin on Pain and Symptoms of Lumbar Spinal Stenosis: A Clinical Trial Study
PICO:
Population - Patients with lumbar spinal stenosis

Intervention - Nasal Calitonin
Comparison - Oral Gabapentin
Outcome - Pain and symptoms

8.4 Title of the Study

The title of the study should have the following elements:

- Outcome
- Population
- Study design
- Place of study

Example 1:

Symptomatic dengue infection during pregnancy and livebirth outcomes in Brazil, 2007–13: a retrospective observational cohort study
   (Lancet Infectious diseases - September 2017, Volume 17, Number 9)

8.5 Introduction

The introduction should have the following components:
- Background of the study
   o   Information about the disease of interest
   o   Current scenario of the disease
- Need for the present study/Rationale for conducting the study
- Page limit

8.6 Review of Literature

Keep in mind the following points:

- Must be exhaustive
  - ➢ Internet search - Google Scholar, Embase, Ovid, Pubmed Central, EBSCO etc.,
  - ➢ Library search
  - ➢ Grey literature (unpublished data)
- Include only recent studies - past 10 years
- Include both national and international studies
- Precise
- Limit in numbers - 10 to 25 studies
- Include Lacunae in literature

How to write??

While writing a review of literature, include the following points:

- Name of the author
- Year of the study
- Place of the study
- Objectives
- Key points in methods
- Results
- Conclusion

8.7 Objectives

The objectives should fulfill SMART criteria.

"SMART"
  S - Specific
  M - Measurable

A - Achievable

R - Realistic

T - Time bound

Example 1:

Quetiapine extended release versus aripiprazole in children and adolescents with first-episode psychosis: the multicentre, double-blind, randomised tolerability and efficacy of antipsychotics (TEA) trial. (LANCET PYSCHIATRY AUGUST 2017)

1. To compare the efficacy and safety of quetiapine-extended release (quetiapine-ER) versus aripiprazole in children and adolescents with first-episode psychosis

2. To determine the differences between quetiapine-extended release and aripiprazole in children and adolescents with first-episode psychosis.

Do these objectives fulfill SMART criteria?

Yes.

8.8 Materials and Methods

Include the following subheadings.

- **Study site**
  - o Place of the study
  - o Describe the place of the study
- **Study design**
  - o Cross-sectional/Case control/Cohort study/ Randomized controlled trial/Quasi-experimental trial
- **Study population** - Cases/Control
  - o Inclusion criteria
  - o Exclusion criteria

- **Study duration**
  - ○ Protocol submission
  - ○ Data collection
  - ○ Total study period
  - ○ Gantt Chart

Figure 8.1 Format (Example 1) of Gantt Chart

Task	Possible start (week)	Length (weeks) min-modal -max	Dependent on task	
1. Preliminary literature search	0	3-4-5		
2. Research question development	0	1-2-3		
3. Methodology development	1	6-8-10		
4. Consideration of ethical requirements	1	1-2-3	3	
5. Ethical approval	3	6-10-14	3,4	
6. Data collection and analysis	9	6-8-10	3,4,5	
7. Write up	2	6-24-26	2,3,4,5,6	
8. Production of final project report	25	1-2-3	7	

Weeks 1 2 3 4 5 6 7 8 9 10 11 12 13 14 15 16 17 18 19 20 21 22 23 24 25 26

Figure 8.2 Format (Example 2) of Gantt Chart

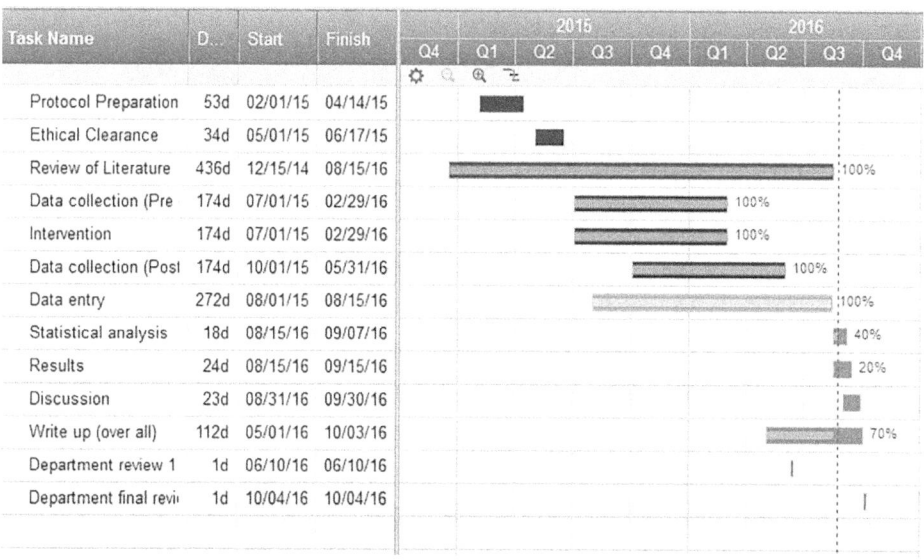

Task Name	D...	Start	Finish	2015 Q4	Q1	Q2	Q3	Q4	2016 Q1	Q2	Q3	Q4
Protocol Preparation	53d	02/01/15	04/14/15									
Ethical Clearance	34d	05/01/15	06/17/15									
Review of Literature	436d	12/15/14	08/15/16								100%	
Data collection (Pre	174d	07/01/15	02/29/16						100%			
Intervention	174d	07/01/15	02/29/16						100%			
Data collection (Post	174d	10/01/15	05/31/16							100%		
Data entry	272d	08/01/15	08/15/16								100%	
Statistical analysis	18d	08/15/16	09/07/16									40%
Results	24d	08/15/16	09/15/16									20%
Discussion	23d	08/31/16	09/30/16									
Write up (over all)	112d	05/01/16	10/03/16								70%	
Department review 1	1d	06/10/16	06/10/16									
Department final revi	1d	10/04/16	10/04/16									

- **Sample size determination**
  - o Formula for calculating sample size
  - o References from previous studies
  - o Name of the software for sample size (if has been used) with version and license
  - o Detailed explanation with substitution of values
  - o Power of the study, alpha error (significance), expected outcome, etc.,

- **Sampling method**
  - o Random/Non-random sample
  - o Justification why such method used

- **Study tool**
  - o Questionnaire structure - Unstructured/semi-structured/fully structured
  - o Intervention - Drug, procedure, surgery/scales
  - o Pretesting and validation details
  - o Brief outline of study proforma

- **Data collection technique**
  - o Recruiting patients
  - o Randomization
  - o Blinding
  - o Procedures/interventions

- **Outcomes of the study**
  - o Primary outcomes
  - o Secondary outcomes

- **Follow up**
  - o Duration of follow up and measurements
  - o Referrals after the study outcome results (if required)

- **Data analysis**
  - Data entry and analysis are done with paid/free/ institutional software
  - Software license number
  - Analysis of variables - quantitative/qualitative
  - Tests of significance that could be applied

8.9 Ethical Committee Approval

  - Ethical committee approval letter details and number

- **Consent**
  - Type of consent/assent obtained
  - Mention about the consent letter

8.10 Working/operative definitions/scales/ intervention procedures

Mention, with references, all the definitions, criteria, and scales used.

8.11 References

Use Vancouver format for journal articles:

Author name(s) - Title of the study - Abbreviated journal name - Month and year - Volume - Issue - Page numbers

Example 1:

Cannon CP, Shah S, Dansky HM, et al. Safety of anacetrapib in patients with or at high risk for coronary heart disease. N Engl J Med 2010;363:2406-15.

8.12 Annexures:

The annexures should include

- ✖ Consent form (English and regional language)
- ✖ Questionnaire/Study proforma (English and regional language)
- ✖ Ethics committee approval forms

9

HOW TO WRITE A CLINICAL CASE REPORT

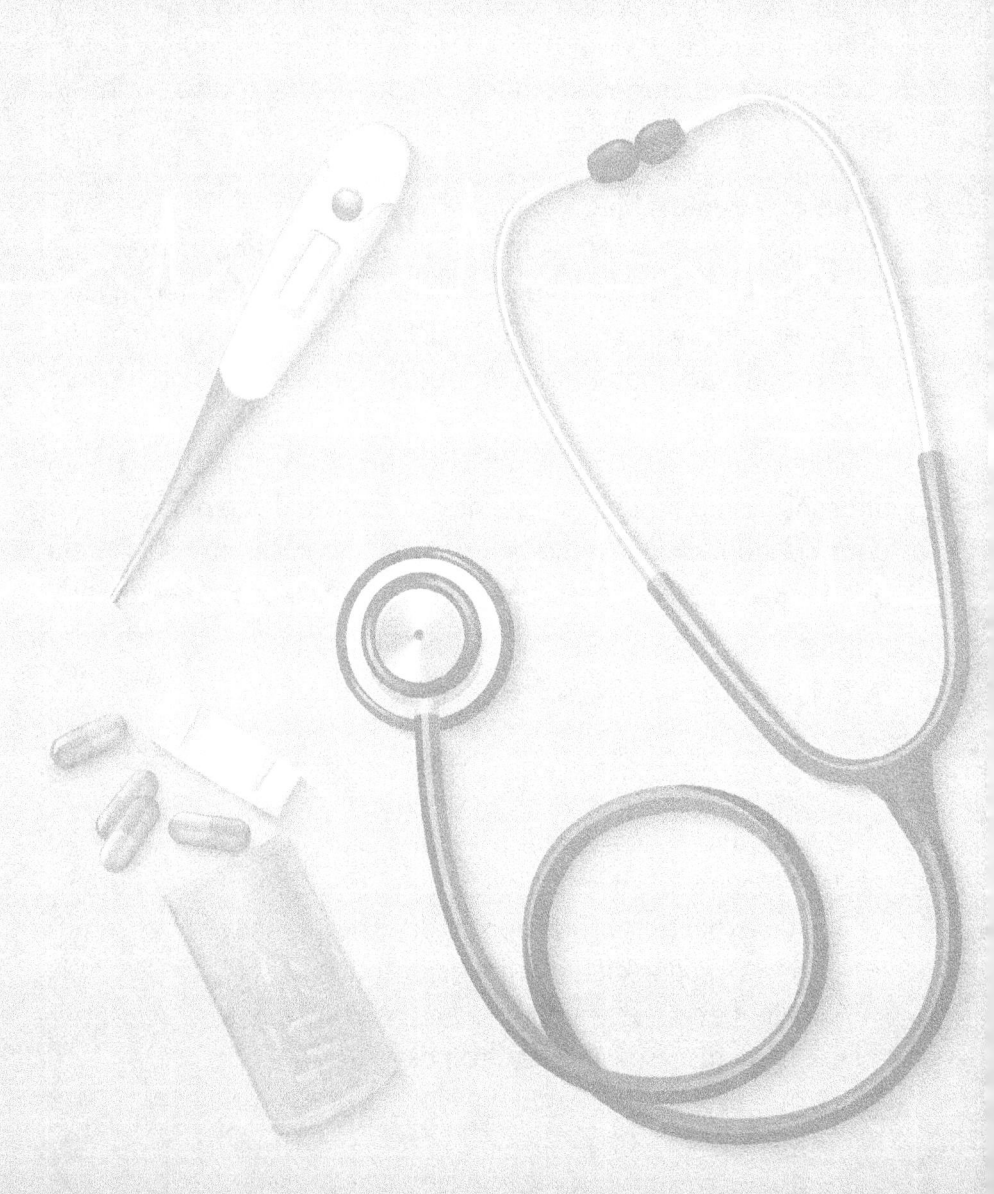

In medical literature, case reports are the first level of evidence. Medical students and working physicians can improve their writing skills by preparing a case report. Their curriculum vitae will look impressive if they submit a case report.

9.1 What is a Case Report?

A case report is a method to share new information gained from clinical practice. It could be a rare medical condition, a novel diagnostic or therapeutic strategy for managing a disease, or an uncommon consequence.

Is the case reportable?

The main objective of reporting a case is to impart new and important knowledge to the medical world. The first step in case report writing is to check medical literature to ensure that the case is new and uncommon. Discussion with experts of the field should be done.

The case should have an uncommon presentation or an unusual combination of events or unusual associations or unusual side effects to therapies. Also, the case may shed light on the novel pathogenesis of a disease or propose a new theory.

9.2 Usefulness of Case Reports

Case reports contribute to our medical knowledge by describing:

1. Unique or nearly unique cases
2. Unexpected events or outcomes (eg. side effects of drugs)
3. Unexpected association of disease parameters
4. New diagnostic techniques or tools
5. New treatment strategies and options
6. New diseases and syndromes

9.3 Steps of Case Report Writing

There are various steps in writing a case report. The steps are as follows:

1. Finding a rare case.
2. Literature search and discussion with the experts of the field.
3. Collecting information related to the case, including consent.
4. Writing discussion and summarizing.
5. Revision and editing.

9.4 Format for a Case Report - Critical Elements

A case report should have the following components:

1. Title
2. Abstract
3. Introduction/Background
4. Literature review
5. Case details
6. Discussion and conclusion
7. References
8. Images if any (Radiological images, histology slides, photographs, etc.)

Before Starting the Write-up

If you work under a department head, you should also obtain permission from the department head or the consultant in charge of the patient's care before submitting your report. This helps in two ways: it ensures that no one else begins writing up the same case, and it allows the expert to provide meaningful and helpful input.

Title
The title of the case report must be precise, informative, and effective.

Abstract
Abstracts should provide an overview of the case and details of the case report. The word limit requirement may vary between journals. Generally, the word limit is around 150-250. The major material of the abstract should be divided into four sections: introduction, case facts, discussion, and conclusion. The format changes with the requirements of the journals.

Introduction
The introduction section should be brief and to the point in order to capture the reader's attention right away. It should be between one and three paragraphs long. It must be written in the present tense. It should have:

1. Background information to get clarity on the subject of discussion
2. Justification that present case is rare – unusual presentation or association
3. Contribution to scientific knowledge

Literature review
This is a very crucial step in the process of case reporting. If a comprehensive search has not been done and the findings have already been reported, there is no novelty of scientific knowledge and it is difficult to publish the article. A literature

review should include the search strategy and scope, as well as the database and keywords searched. Popular search engines include PubMed, Medline, Ovid, EBSCO, Embase, and Google Scholar. Some popular case report journals that are not indexed in PubMEd should be checked as well. For example, International Medical Case Reports Journal.

Case details

This is one of the most important sections of the case report that has the case details. The case is told in a straightforward and enjoyable manner. In order to establish the case's validity, sufficient details must be provided. The general approach, in the absence of headings, is to describe the history, examination findings, investigations, and treatment in that order. Relevant histories must be narrated in detail.

Only the most important positive and negative findings from each stage of the clinical evaluation should be mentioned, with no unnecessary details. While describing the case report, ensure that the causal and temporal relationships are maintained.

At the time of the report, provide detailed descriptions of the treatment's effect, any unexpected side effects, the patient's final outcome, any additional proposed treatments, and the patient's current status. Relevant positive or negative laboratory results, as well as the laboratory's reference range, must be provided. A summary of diagnostic procedures should be provided.

Discussion

Because a well-written discussion and argument will persuade a journal that your case report is worthy of publication, this is the selling point of any case report. The discussion should assess the accuracy, validity, and uniqueness of the patient's case, as well as compare and contrast the case report to previously published literature. The author must ensure the accuracy of the data presented and establish a temporal and causal relationship to ensure the case report's validity. The differences between expected and observed outcomes should be discussed. Alternative explanations and newer hypotheses must be developed. The author should summarize the key findings, make recommendations and draw conclusions.

Conclusion

A clear and justified conclusion should be drawn based on the scientific evidence mentioned in the discussion section. It should include future research opportunities. It is necessary to make a justifiable, evidence-based recommendation. This section should be brief and no more than one paragraph long.

Referencing style

References should be listed in the journal's preferred format. (e.g., Vancouver, Harvard, etc.). The most common referencing style is the Vancouver style. Ideally, the number of references should be limited to ten and only relevant references should be quoted.

Images

Images relevant to the case could be submitted along with the manuscript and such images will keep the reader engaged. Images include histopathological slides, roentgenograms, electrocardiographs, scan images, and other lab tests. Images of skin lesions, ulcers, and other anatomical parts could be used. Any identifying features in the patient's photographs must be removed.

9.5 Order of Writing

The standard order of writing a case report is as follows:

1. Case
2. References
3. Introduction/background
4. Discussion
5. Abstract
6. Title

Foremost, details of the case must be written. Next, references to the literature used in the introduction or background need to be provided, followed by a discussion and conclusion. The abstract must be written after the main content of the manuscript is finalized. It is a good practice to write the title at last.

9.6 Consent issues

As with the other research studies, the confidentiality of the patient needs to be maintained. Any identifying information of the patient should not be revealed. Every effort should be made to maintain the anonymity of the patients. In rare cases, if there is any doubt that anonymity cannot be maintained, written informed consent should be obtained.

Some journals archive consent forms themselves; others require authors to archive consent forms. The format for informed consent must have the following words:

"I understand that the material will be published without my name attached and every attempt will be made to ensure my anonymity. I understand, however, that complete anonymity cannot be guaranteed. It is possible that somebody somewhere – perhaps, for example, someone who looked after me if I was in the hospital, or perhaps a relative – may identify me."

9.7 Writing Tips

While writing manuscripts following do's and don'ts must be kept in mind:

1. Always remember space requirements, i.e., word limits for full article and abstract. The word limit varies with different journals. For instance, the word limit for a full article case report is <2000 for the New England Journal of Medicine.
2. Use appropriate words to describe the conditions.
3. Never use flowery language, remember this is scientific writing.
4. Word limit per sentence should be <20.
5. Use verbs early in the sentence and avoid weak verbs like "to be", "to have".
6. Don't treat patients as commodities. For example, instead of writing "We managed patients with penicillin", write "We managed patients' illness with penicillin" or "We treated patients with penicillin".
7. Don't blame patients for their conditions. For example, instead of writing "Patient was a treatment failure", write "Patient did not respond to treatment".
8. Don't define patients by their disease. For example, instead of writing "diabetics", "arthritics", etc., write "Patient with diabetes", "Patient with arthritis", etc.
9. Avoid using emotionally charged words like "suffered from" or "complained of". Use "had", "reported", etc.

9.8 Authorship Etiquettes

The number of authors should be limited in case reports. The number should be limited to four. All the authors should have contributed to the writing of the manuscripts. All the authors should have approved the final manuscript before submitting it to the journals.

9.9 Journal Selection

While choosing a journal for submission of your case report, consider the following factors:

1. Field
2. Impact factor
3. Likelihood of publication
4. Sample of published case reports

Find three to four suitable journals and review the instructions for authors including word limits. Most case reports will require at least one or two revisions after they are submitted to a journal.

9.10 Reasons for rejections

Some of the reasons for the rejection of case reports for publication are as follows:

1. Unoriginal observation and lack of uniqueness of the case. To avoid this, do a thorough literature search.
2. Poor writing and sweeping generalization.
3. Lack of mention about clinical implications and prospects of future research.

Don't get dejected if your paper is rejected for publication. Try to incorporate changes suggested by reviewers and inputs from experts. Persistence often pays off!

9.11 Checklist for submission of case reports for publication (some items may not be applicable to all case reports)

I. Abstract

- ❑ Introduction/background
- ❑ Case details
- ❑ Discussion
- ❑ Conclusion

II. Introduction

- ❑ Provide background information
- ❑ Describe the case report's purpose.
- ❑ Describe the strategy for the literature review.

Keep your introduction brief and not more than three paragraphs.

III. Case details

- ❑ Only include pertinent patient demographics (age, sex, race, occupation, height, and weight).
- ❑ Describe the patient's complaint as well as his or her current and previous medical histories.
- ❑ Make a record of the patient's medical and family history.
- ❑ List the patient's medication history, including the drug's name, strength, dosage form, route, and dates of administration.

❑ Describe any relevant physical examination findings.
❑ Provide relevant laboratory values to back up your case, as well as reference ranges.
❑ Mention any relevant diagnostic procedure specifics.

Photographs of roentgenograms, electrocardiograms, histopathology, skin lesions, or anatomy relevant to the case are encouraged.

IV. Discussion

❑ Explain or justify the case report's and the literature's similarities and differences.
❑ List the case report's limitations and explain their significance.
❑ To determine the validity of the case report, use a scale such as the Naranjo nomogram.

V. Conclusion

❑ Make evidence-based recommendations and provide a clear and justified conclusion.

Make a list of potential future research areas.

10

HOW TO WRITE AN ORIGINAL ARTICLE

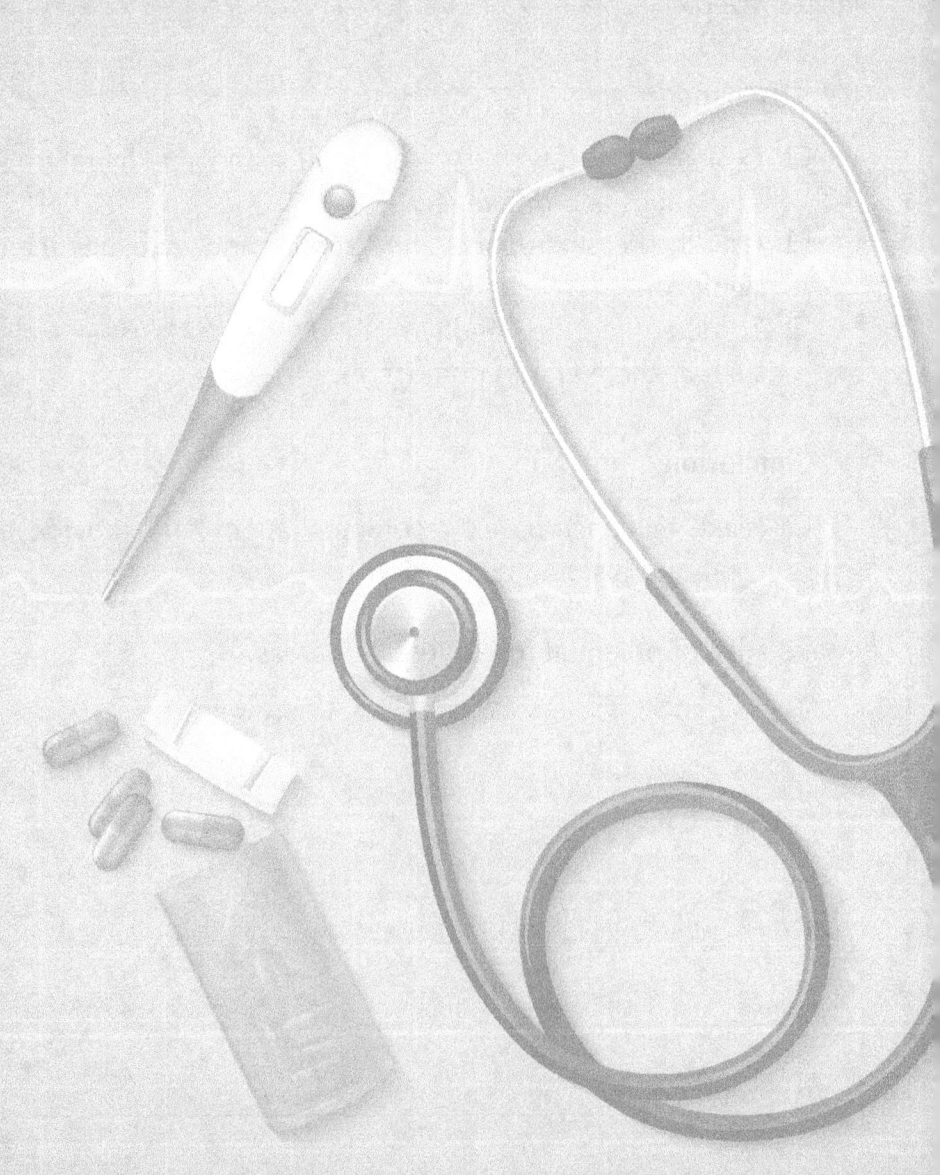

A well-written original article explains what was done, why it was done, how it was done, the outcome of the work, and the relevance of the work.

10.1 Recommended Order for Writing an Original Manuscript

Following order should be followed in writing an original article after finishing the data collection and analysis.

1. Tables and figures
2. Results
3. Methods
4. Introduction
5. Discussion
6. Abstract

10.2 Tables and Figures

Why are tables and figures important?

- Your story's base is made out of tables and figures!
- Titles, abstracts followed by tables and figures may be the first (and possibly only) elements that editors, reviewers, and readers look at!

Tips on tables and figures

- Figures and tables should be able to communicate a whole story on their own. There should be no need for the reader to return to the main text.
- Tell the story with the fewest possible figures and tables.
- Don't include the same information in a figure and a table.

Tables vs. Figures

Figures give:

- Aesthetic appeal
- Display patterns and trends
- Make up a fast story
- Recount the entire story
- Emphasize a certain outcome

Tables give:

- Accurate figures
- Display a large number of values/variables

10.2.1 Table construction

1. **Table title**
   - Determine the table's specific topic or point of discussion.
   - In the table title, column headings, and text of the document, use the same key terms.
   - Keep it short and sweet!

Example 1:

Descriptive characteristics of the two treatment groups, means ± SD or N (%)

2. **Table footnotes**
   - Use superscript symbols to denote footnotes in accordance with journal requirements. A usual sequence is *, †,‡,¶,#,**,††, etc.

o   Explain statistically significant differences with footnotes. For example, *p.01 vs. control by ANOVA.
o   Elaborate abbreviations or explain experiment details in footnotes. For example, The Eating Disorder Inventory.
o   Amenorrhea was described as a lack of 0-3 menstrual cycles each year.

3. **Table format**
    *   Create your tables using tables that have previously been published! Re-inventing the wheel is a waste of time!!
    *   The majority of journals employ three horizontal lines: one line above the column titles, one below the column headings, and one beneath the data.

Note the three horizontal lines in the table shown below:

Variable	Control (n=82)	Intervention (n=82)	P
Age, mean±SD	60.54±8.74	61.42±9.84	0.547
Gender, n (%)			
Male	15 (18.3)	13 (15.9)	0.836
Female	67 (81.7)	69 (84.1)	
Amount of anti-hypertensive medicine consumed, mean±SD	1.29±1.22	1.04±0.77	0.373
Systolic blood pressure , mean±SD	149.94±11.57	154.60±20.11	0.173
Diastolic blood pressure , mean±SD	91.46±4.81	92.66±11.01	0.299
Diabetes mellitus, n (%)	5 (6.1)	6 (7.3)	0.350
Using alternative medicine, n (%)	25 (30.5)	19 (23.2)	0.378
Aware of hypertension, n (%)	60 (73.2)	69 (84.1)	0.127
Family history of hypertension, n (%)	25 (30.5)	60 (73.2)	0.000

Data were presented as n (%) or mean±SD. SD: Standard deviation

*   Follow journal-specific guidelines:
    o   Arabic or Roman numerals
    o   Table number, title, column, headings, and data should be centered or flush left
    o   Italics and capital letters
    o   The positioning of footnotes
    o   The nature of footnote symbols

Nuggets

For making tables, following points need to be remembered:

- Three horizontal lines

- Remove grid lines!

- Double-check that everything is in order and looks professional!

- In decimals, use a suitable amount of significant digits.

- Mention units!

- Remove columns that aren't needed.

10.2.2 Figures:

1. Primary evidence

- Photographs, pathology slides, X-rays, electron micrographs, gels, etc.
- Indicates data quality

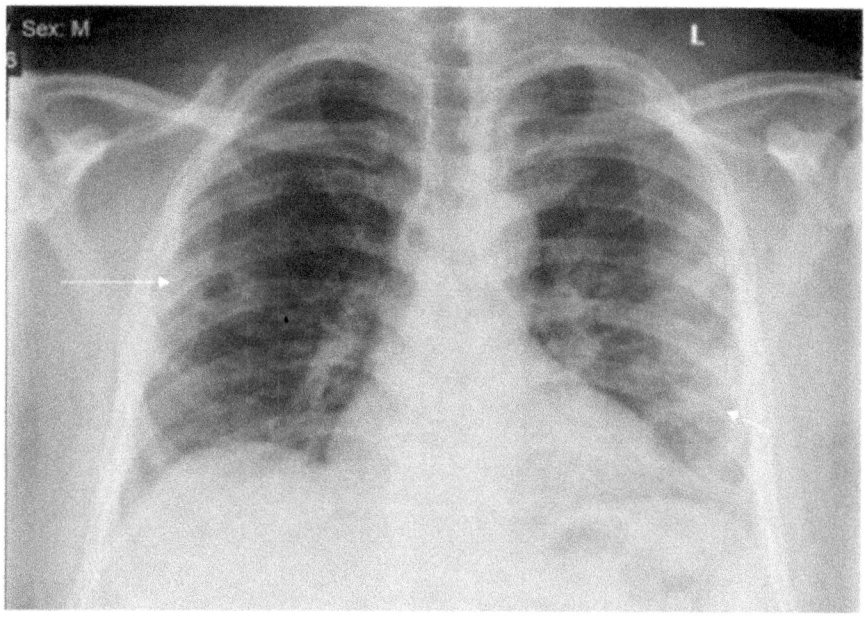

Image 1 Chest X-ray of a COVID-19 positive patient. The atoll sign (long arrow) of organized pneumonia can be seen in the right mid-zonal lesion with central lucency. Small air space consolidation opacities with reticular thickening were detected in the lower zone of the left (short arrow).

Figure Legends
Self-explanatory. May contain:
1. 1. Short title
2. 2. Crucial experimental details
3. 3. Symbol or line/bar pattern definitions
4. 4. Panel explanation (A, B, C, D, etc.)Statistical information (tests used, p-values, etc.)

2. Graphs
- Bar graphs, line graphs, histograms, scatter plots, boxplots, survival curves, etc.

Line Graphs

- Can be used to demonstrate patterns over time, age, or dose.
- May show group or individual averages

Line Diagram	Pie Chart

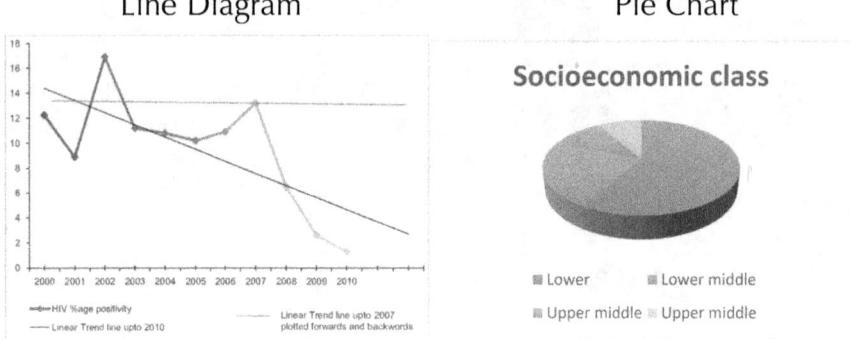

Bar Graph

- Used to compare groups at a single moment in time
- Conveys a brief visual story

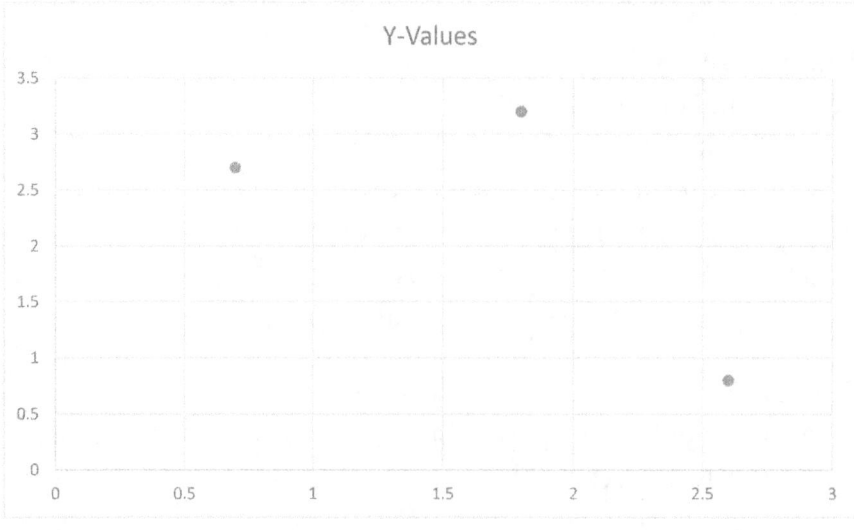

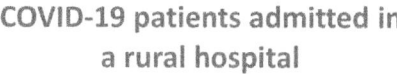

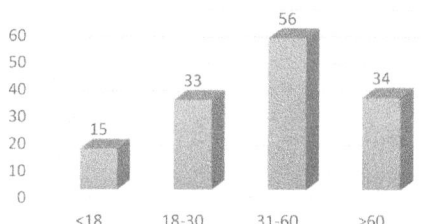

Scatter plots

- It's a diagram that depicts the relationship between any two quantitative variables (particularly linear correlation)
- Enables the reader to see individual data, resulting in more information

Scatter plot

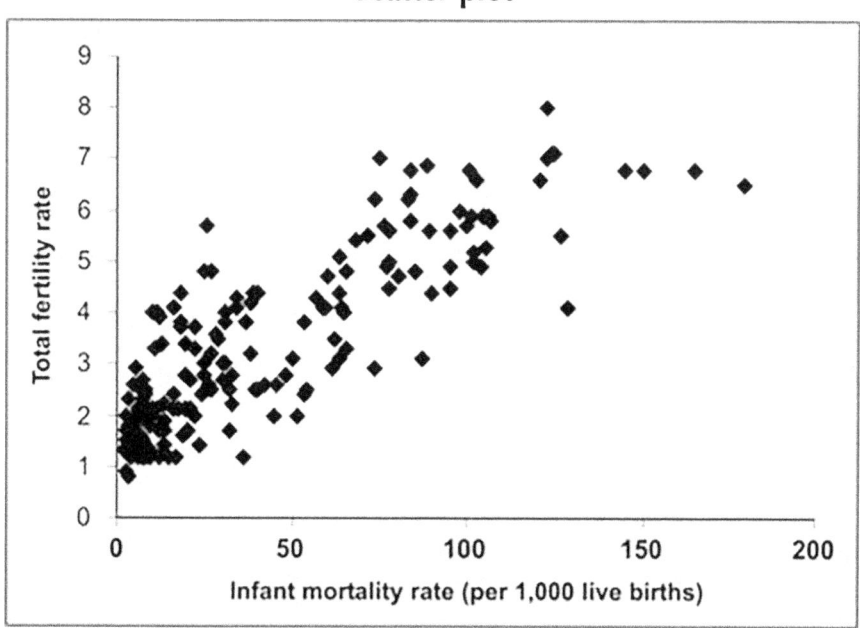

Nuggets

Tips for Graphs

- Tell a quick visual story.

- Keep it simple!

- Make it easy to distinguish groups (e.g., triangles vs. circles vs. squares is not easy!)

- If it's too complicated, put it in a table.

3. Drawings and diagrams

- Exemplify an experimental setup or workflow
- Show the flow of participants
- Show cause and effect linkages or cycles
- Propose a hypothetical model
- Use cartoons to portray microscopic particles or microorganisms

10.3 Results

Results = NOT raw data
The results section should:

- Highlight simple relationships
- Summarize what the data shows
- Explain long-term trends
- Include supporting data in the form of figures or tables.

Principles for writing results

- Use headers to divide the section into subsections (if needed)
- Add to the information currently shown in the tables and figures.
- Provide specific values that are not depicted in the figure.
- If the table contains absolute figures, report the percent change or percent difference.
- Only the most important numbers should be highlighted or repeated. Avoid simply mentioning the numbers that can also be found in tables and figures.
- Don't forget to discuss negative and control outcomes.
- The term "significant" should only be used for statistically significant entities.
- Keep the information about what you did for the methods section to yourself.
- Do not, for example, discuss the rationale for statistical analyses in the Results section.
- Save your comments on the significance of your findings for the discussion section. Use the active voice.
  - o More lively!
  - o Because you can discuss the subjects of your experiments, "we" can be used sparingly while keeping the active voice!

Which verb tense do I use?

Past tense

For completed actions, use the past tense.

As an example, We found that...

Females were more likely to...

Women smoked fewer cigarettes than...

Present tense
Use the present tense for assertions that remain true, for example, what the tables show, what you believe, and what the data imply. For instance,

Figure 1 shows...
The findings confirm...
The data suggest...
We believe that this shows...

10.4 Methods

Principles for writing methods:

- Provide a concise picture of what was accomplished.
- Provide enough information for the study to be replicated (like a recipe!).
- Be thorough, yet make your reader's life easier!
- Use subheadings to divide the document into smaller pieces.
- For regularly used approaches, cite a source.
- If possible, show the information in a flowchart or table.
- In the Methods section, you may utilize the passive voice and jargon more freely.

Pro tips:

- Make your reader's life easier.
- Break into sub-sections with informative subheadings.
- Use flow diagrams or tables to help simplify explanations of methods!

> ## Nuggets
> Methods should answer - Who, what, when, where, how, and why...?

10.5 Introduction

About Introduction

- The good news is that writing the introduction is simpler than you think!
- Follows a fairly standard format
- Typically three paragraphs in length
- The recommended paragraph length is 2 to 5 paragraphs.
- It should not be an exhaustive review of your general topic; rather, it should concentrate on the hypothesis or goal of your study.

Inverted cone approach:

For writing, the introduction section follows an inverted cone approach.

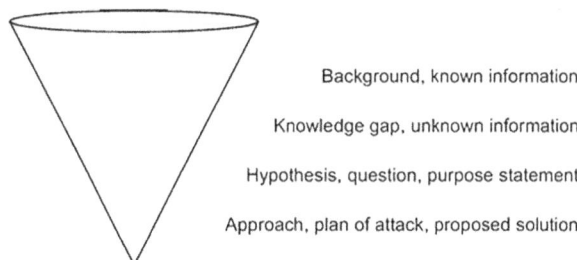

Background, known information

Knowledge gap, unknown information

Hypothesis, question, purpose statement

Approach, plan of attack, proposed solution

Outline of Introduction section:

1) What is unknown?
2) What is known?

3) Previous research gaps and limitations
4) Your most pressing question/hypothesis/goal
5) Your experimental strategy
6) Explain why your study experiment is novel/unique, distinct, and significant (fills any scientific gaps)

These contents correspond to roughly three paragraphs.

Tips for writing the Introduction section:

- Keep paragraphs short.
- Write for a broad audience by being clear, non-technical, and concise.
- Lead the reader from the known to the unknown. Finally, pose your specific query. (Known)
- Highlight how your research fills in the gaps. (The unidentified)Explicitly state your research question/aim/hypothesis
  - "We asked whether"; "Our hypothesis was"; "We tested the hypothesis that"; "Our aim/s was/were"
- Do not answer the research question (no results or implications).
- Summarize at a high level! Leave detailed descriptions, speculations, and criticisms of particular studies for the Discussion section.

10.6 Discussion

What is discussion?

- Is the most difficult to write
- Provides you with the greatest amount of freedom

Gives you the most opportunities to showcase your writing.

Upright the cone!

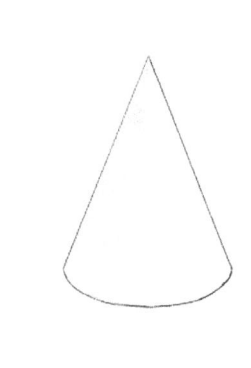	<ul><li>Respond to the question.</li><li>Back up your claim (your data, data from others)</li><li>Defend your conclusion (prepare for criticism)</li><li>Provide the "big picture" take-home message- what do my findings mean and why should anyone bother?</li></ul>

Tips to write Discussion section

- Showcase good writing!
- Use the active voice.
- Tell it like a story.
- Start and end with the main finding "We found that…".
- Don't travel too far from your data.
- Focus on what your data do prove, not what you had hoped your data would prove.
- Focus on the limitations that matter, not generic limitations.
- Make sure your take-home message is clear and consistent.

What Not To Do!

Do not begin your discussion in this manner.:!

There are several limitations to this meta-analysis. The estimates of melanoma risk after using sunlamps/sunbeds are based on data published in a series of ten articles over a 20-year period. A pooled analysis of the 10 studies' original observations would have provided a more powerful approach.

Which tense to use?

Past

When referring to details of the study, results, analyses, and background.

- Subjects might have experienced
- Sharma S et al. found
- We found that

Present

When talking about what the data suggest.

- Possible I explanations include
- The greater bone loss suggests
- The reason for this discrepancy is unclear.

10.7 Abstract

- Is a synopsis of the main plot
- Highlights key points from each section of the paper
- Is typically 100-300 words long
- Can stand on its own
- Is used in electronic search engines, along with the title
- Most of the time, the only part that people read is the introduction.

Elements of abstract:

- Background
  - Research question/objectives
  - "We inquired whether", "We speculated that,"...

- Experiment(s)
- A brief synopsis of materials and methods
- Results
  - Important findings
  - Very little simple data

- Conclusion
  - The response to the question posed/the take-home message
  - Inference, supposition, or recommendation

11

CRITICAL APPRAISAL OF
A RESEARCH ARTICLE

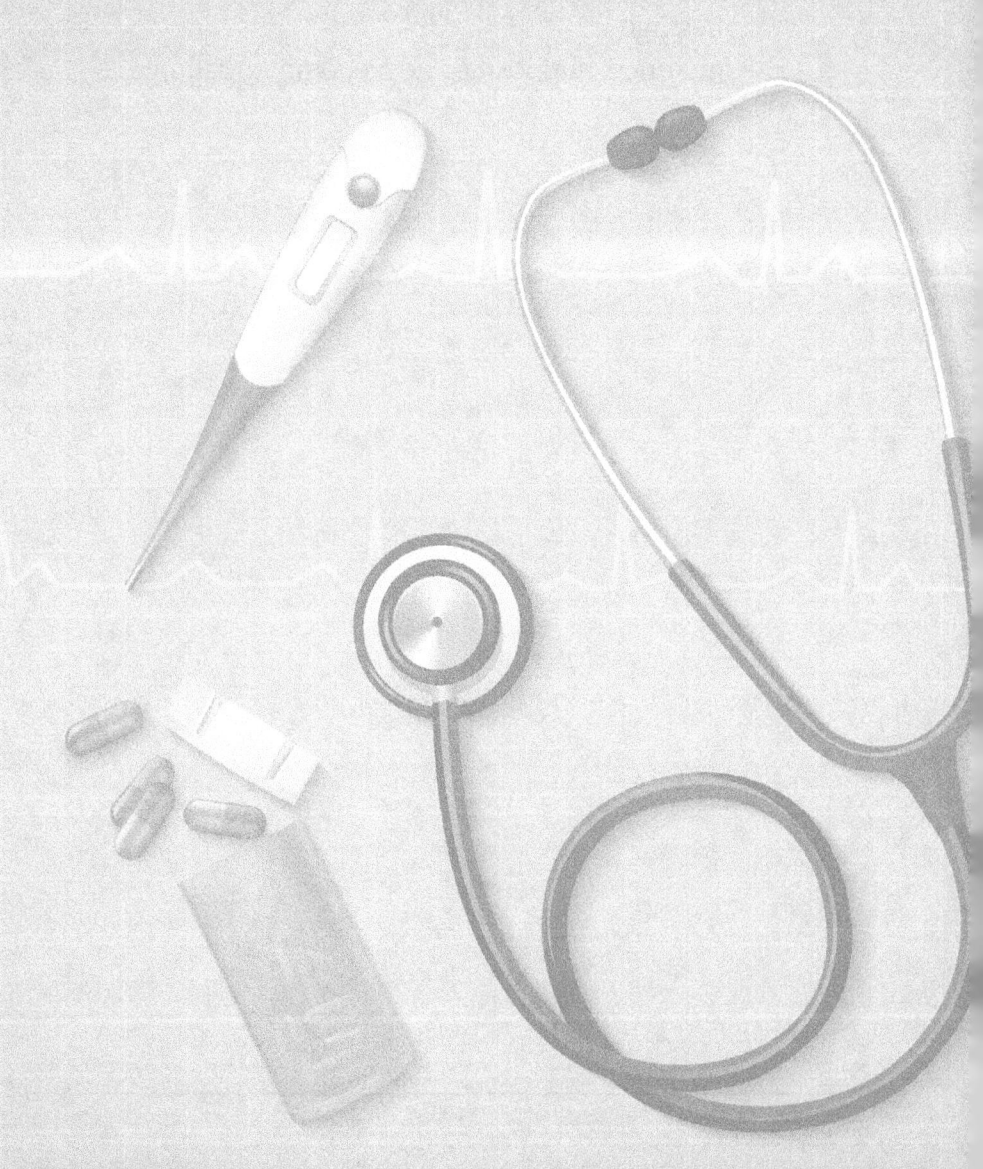

Critical appraisal is defined as the "...application of rules of evidence to a study to assess the validity of the data, completeness of reporting, methods and procedures, conclusions, compliance with ethical standards, etc. The rules of evidence vary with circumstances."

- J E Last

A systematic process for identifying one's strengths and weaknesses of a research article is known as critical appraisal. The key components of critical appraisal are assessing the appropriateness of the study design for the research question and assessing the study's methodological aspects.

11.1 Why Critically Appraise an Article?

Practicing evidence-based medicine requires a few steps:

1. Search for the best available evidence
2. Appraisal of the evidence critically for validity and reliability
3. Application of the evidence in clinical decision-making process

The clinical decision-making process is required at two levels - 1. Handling an individual patient and 2. Deciding standard treatment guidelines for a group of patients with a disease. For both levels, appraising the published article critically helps in decision making.

Also, there is an escalating increase in the number of new medical research articles published annually - more than 12,000 new articles are added to the MEDLINE database every week.

Clinicians can manage this 'information overload' by developing skills in critical appraisal, which helps them to focus only on high-quality studies and extrapolate the studies to their clinical practice.

As a result, a critical appraisal provides clinicians with a foundation for deciding whether to use the findings of a study in daily clinical practice.

11.2 Guidelines for Critical Appraisal of Various Study Designs

Study type	Guidelines
Observational studies	STROBE
Randomized controlled trials	CONSORT
Systematic reviews and meta-analyses of intervention studies	PRISMA, QUOROM, AMSTAR, CASP
Systematic reviews and meta-analyses of observational studies	MOOSE
Nonrandomized evaluations of behavioral and public health interventions	TREND
Diagnostic studies	STARD, TRIPOD
Microarray studies	MIAME
Qualitative studies	COREQ, SRQR
Case reports	CARE
Economic evaluations	CHEERS
Quality improvement studies	SQUIRE
Animal preclinical studies	ARRIVE
Study protocols	SPIRIT, PRISMA-P

11.3 Critical Appraisal Process

1. Authors

Look at the authors' credentials and their background. Some information or lack of it may give a warning sign about the study's integrity. The Journal name and impact factor of the journal does not guarantee the trustworthiness of the study results. Mistakes and errors do occur in high-quality journals with great impact factors too. Contact details of corresponding authors must be provided.

2. Title and abstract

The title should be clear, concise and should indicate the type of study design. If the study is a randomized control trial, the word "randomized" should be used in the title. The abstract section should provide a balanced summary of what was done and what was found. Some readers use abstracts to screen articles before deciding whether to read the complete article. The abstract should not contain information not found in the body of the paper and should accurately represent what is found in the full article. In the case of randomized trials, the details of the harm should also be mentioned in the abstract, as failure to do so may lead to a misinterpretation of the trial results. According to the revised CONSORT statement, there is a list of essential items that authors should include in their reporting abstract. Journals have their unique reporting format, word limits, and structure. CONSORT, on the other hand, recommends a list of items to include in the abstract.

Background

Scientific background and rationale for conducting the study have to be explained. A gap in the literature and the present study's role in adding information to the scientific world needs to be explained. The rationale could be explanatory (for example, to assess a drug's potential impact on liver function) or pragmatic (for instance, to guide practice by comparing the potential benefits of two treatments).

Authors should provide a plausible explanation for the benefits of the intervention and report any negative effects of such active interventions. According to the Helsinki Declaration, biomedical research involving humans should be based on a thorough scientific literature search.

3. Hypotheses/Objectives

Hypotheses are very specific questions being tested to see if they can help meet the objectives. The study should state specific objectives, including any pre-specified hypotheses.

4. Methods

Study design

The study design and its key elements should be clearly mentioned. In RCT, the type of trial – superiority, non-inferiority, or equivalence trial should be defined. Study designs in RCT can be two-arm parallel, multi-arm parallel, cross over, cluster, and factorial designs. In few RCTs, the study design is not determined at the start of the trial-adaptive design. It is usually a multistage study design that uses the data collected to decide some modifications without affecting the study's validity and integrity. The modifications incorporated are usually in the number of arms and sample sizes. However, there are ethical, practical, and statistical issues with such designs.

Study setting

Study setting, location of study conduction, period of recruitment or data collection, follow-up, and time frames should be mentioned. Information about the study setting is crucial to determine the generalizability of the study findings. Any other information about the study settings that have an influence on the observed results, such as problems with transportation affecting the participation or delays, need to be mentioned.

Study sample

A comprehensive description of the selection criteria of the study participants should be made as it is central to the external validity of the study. Exclusion of some persons due to influence in affecting results by their baseline characteristics or vulnerability to harm from study intervention is mentioned.

In RCT, the type of randomization done (simple, restricted, blocked, stratified, or minimization), allocation ratio, and number of participants in each arm should be clearly mentioned. Blinding type (single, double, or triple) and allocation concealment mechanisms must be reported. Mention the persons involved in allocation, enrollment, and assigning participants to interventions.

Quantitative variables

Defining all the variables – outcomes, exposure and potential confounders, and effect modifiers and criteria, if used – should be mentioned. Methods of assessment (measurements) and their standardization should be mentioned. Description of comparability of assessment methods, if there is more than one group, should be done.

Interventions

In drug intervention, name of the drug, dose, timing and duration of administration, and route of administration of all the arms of the study should be described in detail. Many trials are conducted for longer periods. Due to ethical concerns, the study may need to be terminated. Details of interim analysis and stopping guidelines should be discussed. It's also a good idea to include the minimum, maximum, and median duration of follow-up.

Outcomes

The number of proposed outcomes for measurement should be included. All outcome measures, both primary or secondary, must be explained in detail. The number of times the outcomes were measured, as well as the primary, co-primary, and secondary endpoints of the study, should be mentioned. Unexpected outcomes or adverse reactions to the intervention should be recorded, whether as a primary or as a secondary outcome.

All major and minor changes or deviations from the protocol, including changes to eligibility criteria, interventions, data collection, and method of analysis, must be reported by the authors. Any changes in trial results that occur after the study begins should be explained.

Sample size

The authors should elaborate on how the sample size was determined. The outcome used for calculating the sample size is mentioned. In RCT, mention the variables required for sample size calculation - 1. Estimated outcomes in each group, 2. Type I error (α), 3. Power of the study (type II error or β), and 4. Standard deviation of the measurement should be done. Ideally, the study size should be large enough to have a high power of detecting a clinically significant difference of a given size as statistically significant, if such a difference exists.

Participants' flow diagram

Participants' flow diagram is strongly recommended in RCT. The number of participants enrolled in each arm after being found eligible, number of participants who underwent randomization, lost to follow-up numbers and numbers included for analysis should be reported in a flow diagram. Reasons for any decrease in number at any phase should be mentioned.

In the majority of follow-up studies, attrition due to loss to follow-up is unavoidable. Other reasons for the drop in the number of participants include ineligibility, withdrawal from treatment, and poor protocol adherence.

Bias reporting

Authors should m all the potential bias of the study. Discussion of bias both in magnitude and direction should be made. Bias could have occurred at recruitment, data collection and analysis levels and these biases should be addressed.

Statistical methods

All statistical methods used should be mentioned. Addressing and handling of missing data should be mentioned. Authors should report which analyses were pre-specified. If subgroup analyses were undertaken, authors should report which subgroups were examined, why, if they were pre-specified, and how many were pre-specified. In RCT, the type of analysis needs to be mentioned - per protocol or intention to treat analysis.

5. Results

Descriptive data details, such as study participant characteristics (e.g., demographic, clinical, social, etc.), as well as information on exposures and potential confounders, should be presented. Outcomes and summary metrics must be mentioned. The risk ratio (relative risk), odds ratio, or risk difference can be used for binary outcomes; the hazard ratio or difference in median survival time can be used for survival time data; and the difference in means is usually used for continuous data. For the contrast between groups, values with confidence intervals should be presented. Unadjusted estimates and unadjusted estimates, as well as their precision, must be reported. Other types of analysis, such as sensitivity analysis, factor analysis, and so on, are also reported.

6. Discussion

It is recommended that the authors should structure the discussion section by presenting 1. Brief description of the key results, 2. Rational justification and explanations, 3. Comparison with a similar picture from previously published studies, 4. Limitations of the present study, and 5. Clinical and research implications of the study findings.

External validity, also known as generalizability or applicability, refers to how well a study's findings can be applied to other situations. The extent to which the trial's design and execution eliminate the possibility of bias is referred to as internal validity. An internally valid study is required for external validity. There should be a discussion about the study's generalizability (external validity), as well as the study's limitations and the methods used to compensate for these limitations.

Different journals have different standard styles of referencing. References should be quoted for all sources cited in the text, tables, and figures of the article. The references cited should help the reader to explore further. All the references should be up to date and new.

7. Conflict of interest

When personal factors have the potential to influence professional roles and responsibilities, a conflict of interest occurs. According to studies, pharmaceutical industry-funded research is more likely to produce results that favor the company's product. Financial conflicts of interest are extremely common and are becoming increasingly recognized in clinical practice and research. The key question here is whether all potential conflicts of interest have been identified and how they have been addressed. One method for dealing with conflicts of interest is open disclosure. The source of funding and the role of the funding agency must be clearly stated. For example, the researchers must state that the funding agency had no influence on the research protocol, data analysis, or findings interpretation.

8. Registration and protocol

International Committee of Medical Journal Editors (ICMJE) recommends registration of the clinical trials before the enrollment of the first participant. The name of the register and the unique registration number of the trial should be provided by the authors. For instance, the trial is listed on clinical trials. gov (Number NCT8888888). Authors should mention the reason if they have not registered their trial.

Also, mention the availability and accessibility of the trial protocol. Some journals publish trial protocols, which can be cited when reporting the main findings of the trial.

9. General considerations

1. Is uniform terminology used throughout the article?? (e.g., Abbreviations and measurement units)

2. Is the flow of the writing smooth, coherent, and understandable?
3. Are the contents of different sections of the paper placed appropriately?

11.4 Key Issues to be Considered for Individual Study Designs

Key issues of methodology to be considered for appraisal in systematic reviews and meta-analyses
✓ Did you include all relevant studies? Has a comprehensive search been done? ✓ Did it exclude any articles based on their language or other characteristics? Has an assessment of publication bias been made? • How was the data extraction done? (by two independent reviewers or not) • Were the patients, interventions, and outcomes of primary studies described? • Was a quality assessment of the primary studies made? • Was the appropriateness of combining results for the purpose of calculating the summary measure evaluated?

Key issues of methodology to be considered for appraisal in randomized controlled trials.
• Was the group assignment procedure truly random? Was there any chance for the participants to know or guess their group allocation? • What was the type of blinding used and how successful was it? • Was an objective assessment of outcomes made? • Were any participants excluded in the final analysis who were allocated into the groups?

Key issues of methodology to be considered for appraisal in a cohort study

- What type of study is it – prospective or retrospective?
- Does the cohort represent the defined population?
- Was identification of all possible confounding factors made?
- Was accurate measurement of exposures, outcomes, and confounding factors made?
- How much proportion was lost to follow-up?
- Was there sufficient follow-up time??

Key issues of methodology to be considered for appraisal in a case-control study

- Was the definition of control-case clear?
- Did the cases represent the defined population?
- Are the controls drawn from the same population as that of cases?
- Were the parameters of the study the same for both cases and controls?
- Was there a chance of recall bias?

Key issues of methodology to be considered for appraisal in a cross-sectional study

- Was the sample of the study taken representative of the study population?
- Was the response rate sufficiently high?
- Was the measurement of exposures, outcomes, and confounding factors made accurately?
- Was there an assessment of the wide range of severity of the disease?

Key issues of methodology to be considered for appraisal in a case study
• How were the cases discovered? Is it better to be prospective or retrospective? • Is the sample of cases representative? • Can you apply the findings in your practice? • Did all relevant exposures, outcomes, and potential confounding factors get measured correctly?

11.5 Appraisal of Qualitative Research

Qualitative Research

Before discussing the critical appraisal of a qualitative study, an overview of the qualitative type of study is mandatory.

Qualitative research is different from quantitative research in various aspects. Data is collected via observations and interviews with an intention to explore the area of interest at first, followed by the generation of a hypothesis from the data. This is called inductive reasoning. The strength of qualitative research lies in its validity or closeness to the truth. A good qualitative study gets to the heart of a topic rather than just skimming the surface. Data triangulation is one method of increasing the validity of methods.

The methods of qualitative research are as follows:

1. Study of documents
2. Passive observation
3. Positive observation
4. Focus group discussion
5. In-depth interviews

Appraisal of a qualitative study

Question 1 Did the study describe addressing clinical problem via a specific question?

The first thing to note in qualitative research, as in quantitative research, is why the research was conducted and what specific question it addressed. Though the definitive research question may not be clearly focused on at the start of a qualitative study, it should have been formulated by the time the report is written.

Question 2 Was a qualitative approach appropriate for the subject of interest?

Qualitative methods were the most appropriate if the objective of research is to explore a deeper understanding of any specific clinical interest. If the objective of the study is to determine incidence of disease, frequency of adverse reactions to drug, testing a cause-effect hypothesis, and comparison of the benefit-risk ratio of two drugs, then qualitative methods are clearly inappropriate.

Question 3 How was the selection of study setting and study subjects done?

In a qualitative study, the sample is selected according to convenience. The sample that seems to be fit for the study will be chosen. The purpose of a qualitative study is to get an in-depth understanding of the views or opinions of either individuals or groups and a sample is deliberately chosen that would be appropriate as the subject of research interest. Appraisal of the appropriateness of study setting and sample needs to be done.

Question 4 What was the researchers' perspective and its influence on data recording?

Data from focus group discussions and semi-structured interviews are likely to be heavily influenced by the interviewer's beliefs about the research statement. This issue could be addressed through interviews with someone who has no opinions and no ideological perspective. It is necessary to ensure that this issue is addressed in the study.

Question 5 What methods do the researcher use for collecting data?

Similar to the sampling strategy, there are no clear-cut criteria about the details to be included in data collection. Appropriateness of the method of data collection in a qualitative study must be assessed.

Question 6 What are the methods used for analyzing the data and the details of quality control measures implemented?

In qualitative research, data analysis must be done methodically rather than simply presenting some "interesting quotes" that support a particular conclusion. Content analysis is a systematic method of data analysis that entails creating a list of coded categories and transcribing each segment of data into these codes. Two or more independent researchers can perform quality control by analyzing and codifying the generated data. Furthermore, some researchers believe that only the person who is most immersed in the fieldwork has genuine insight into the meaning of the data.

Question 7 What about the credibility of the results?

In contrast to quantitative studies, we cannot judge the credibility of the results based on precision, accuracy, significance with confidence intervals, or the number needed to treat. More than just common sense is required to determine whether the results are credible and reasonable, as well as their implications.

Question 8 Are the findings transferable?

Though there are criticisms about the generalizability of the study findings to other settings, the theoretical sampling frame used in the qualitative study is better in transferability of results than the convenience sampling method of quantitative studies.

11.6 Reporting Guidelines

There are reporting guidelines for different study designs. These are available online.

List of Guidelines

- STROBE
- CONSORT
- QUOROM
- MOOSE
- PRISMA P
- CHEERS
- SRQR
- CARE

12

PEER REVIEWING

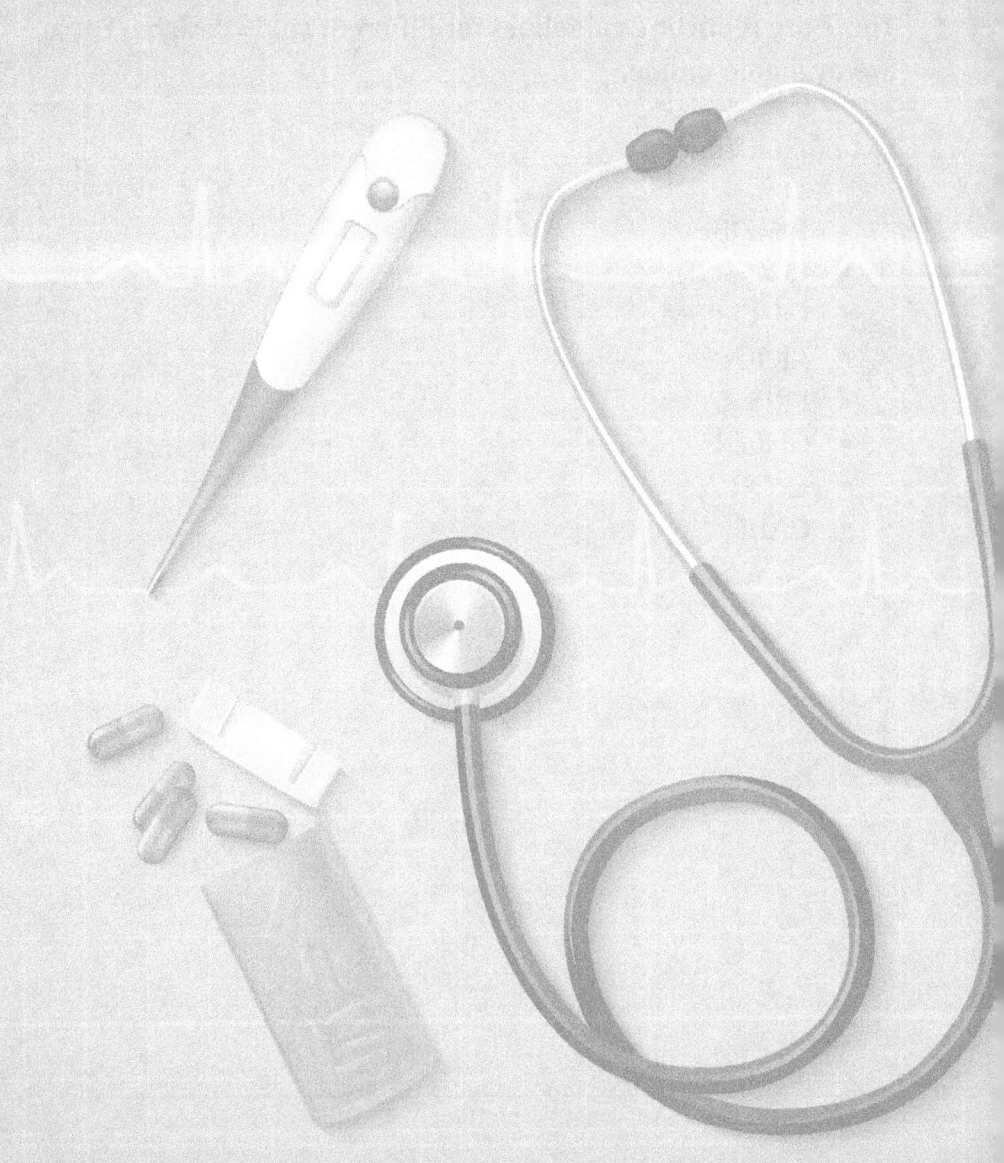

12.1 What is Peer Reviewing?

Peer review is the process of evaluating work by one or more persons who have similar skills to the work's creators (peers). It serves as a means for competent members of a profession to self-regulate within the relevant field. To maintain quality standards, increase performance, and offer credibility, peer review procedures are used.

12.1 Types of Peer Review

The types of peer reviewing process are as follows:

Single-blind
The most prevalent type of blind review is when authors are unaware of the reviewers' identities.

Double-blind
The writers are also hidden from reviewers.

Open
Reviewers and authors are not blinded and the names of the reviewers (and their reviews) may be made public.

Peer review after publication
Blogs, online comments, and other forms of online communication are all examples of this type of peer review.

More formal post-publication vetting techniques may become available in the near future.

12.3 Process

1. Look over the abstract.

2. Go straight to the data.

- First, go over both the tables and figures.
- Make your judgments.
- Are the figures and tables self-contained?
- Are there any statistical inconsistencies?
- Is there any information that is repeated?

3. Go over the page once more.

- Are the writers' conclusions consistent with their data?
- Is the paper well-written or did you have trouble getting through it?
- It shouldn't be necessary for you to battle!

4. Is the document's length justified in light of the amount of new information provided by the data? **Read the introduction carefully.**

- Is it short and sweet enough?
- Is it like this: known->unknown->research question/ hypothesis?
- Is the study's hypotheses or goals stated clearly?
- Is there any additional information about the project that should be included in the methods?
- Is there any information about what was discovered that you believe should be included in the results?
- Is there any material about prior research or mechanisms that are distracting and not directly related to the

hypothesis being investigated? If this is the case, it should be moved to the section for discussion.

- Do the authors describe the gaps in the literature that they are attempting to fill?

5. **Check out the methods carefully.**

- Read through this section to find answers to your data-related questions. Was everything objectively measured or subjectively measured? What were the instruments used?
- Is the study flawed in some way, such as the lack of a control group?
- Pay close attention to the data part.

6. Study the results diligently.

- Study this section while looking at the tables as well as figures.
- Does each section include a table or figure that closely corresponds to it?
- Do the authors summarize the table's primary trends and topics, or do they simply repeat what's there?
- If graphs are used, do the authors provide precise numerical values in the text if they are not shown in the graph?
- Are the authors telling the truth, or are they directing your attention to what they want you to see?
- Do the authors exaggerate statistical significance by ignoring the magnitude of the effect or the fact that many subgroup analyses were performed?
- Is this a lengthy section?

7. Scrutinize each table and figure.

- Did the authors use the most relevant statistics?
- Is the same story being told by more than one table or figure? Table 1 displays the mean values for the two groups as well as the statistical significance determined by a test. Table 2 shows the confidence intervals for mean differences for the same data.
- Is there evidence of deliberate cherry-picking or omission of data?
- Are any graphs deceptive in any way, such as by manipulating the area or axes?
- Is a proper control/placebo group always present in comparison to the "treatment" group?
- Are there any inconsistencies in the data shown from one table to the next?
- Did the writers make any mistakes when transferring data from tables/results to the abstract?

8. Read the discussion carefully.

- Is it clear and simple to state what was discovered and what is new in the first paragraph?
- Do the writers' conclusions make sense or do they go too far?
- Do they differentiate between hypothesis-driven and exploratory conclusions?
- Is the writing clear and concise (use only active voice!)?
  Is there any sort of order or pattern to their conversation, or are they just going around in circles?
- Is it possible to condense the discussion?

- Did they address the issues that you're concerned about? (as opposed to arbitrary constraints imposed for the sake of having some)
- Are the references they cite up to date?
- Have they left out any important references?

12.4 Comments to Authors

- Begin with a one-paragraph "overview". Describe what you believe to be the work's most important discovery and significance.
- Make two or three encouraging, positive comments about the work. Is the writing good, for example, if the methods are questionable? Is the research question particularly interesting or novel? (For example, "This is an intriguing manuscript with several strengths.", "The authors should be applauded for…", "The discovery that XX is significant…", etc.)
- Identify a few major limitations in the design, writing/ presentation, or conclusions of the study. (For example, "The study is limited because there is no control group.", "The overall writing or presentation could be better.", "The authors' findings may have been exaggerated.", "The paper's conclusions are based on shaky evidence.", "The study is exploratory rather than hypothesis-driven.", etc.)
- Avoid disclosing your overall recommendation to the authors (rejection/acceptance).
- Highlight specific errors.
- Make a list of the problems you discovered during your review.
- Make specific revision suggestions.

Key considerations:

- The first one will take a long time to complete. As you progress, you will become increasingly faster at these. Review others in the same way that you would like to be reviewed!
- Assume the other side is some poor graduate student who did all the work and whose self-esteem and career are dependent on your feedback. Do not "lecture" the authors. For example, "The authors should delete table 5; not only is it completely irrelevant, but it also reveals their utter lack of statistical understanding."
- Instead, present your recommendations as suggestions. For example, "Table 5 contains unnecessary information (for example…), and a Pearson's correlation coefficient may not be appropriate here. The authors should consider revising or omitting the table."
- Tone is important!
- Do not criticize the authors! Examine the work for flaws.
- Avoid broad generalizations; instead, point out specific mistakes.
- When possible, prefer to use positive rather than negative language: "The paper is poorly written." vs. "The writing and presentation could be improved."

12.5 Comments to Editors (authors don't see these):

- Fill out the journal "assessment sheet" (this varies with the journals).
- Give the recommendation:
  - o Accept
  - o Accept with minor revisions

- o Reject with the opportunity to revise
- o Reject

- Provide the editors with a succinct overall statement that justifies your ranking. Be open and honest with the editors about your thoughts and concerns.

Nuggets: Reviewer = NOT Copy Editor

Don't waste your time nitpicking.

Concentrate on the big picture.

If the manuscript contains more copy-editing errors, mention this in general terms and provide 1 or 2 examples. e.g. "The manuscript contains typos, such as..."

13

GAME OF PUBLISHING

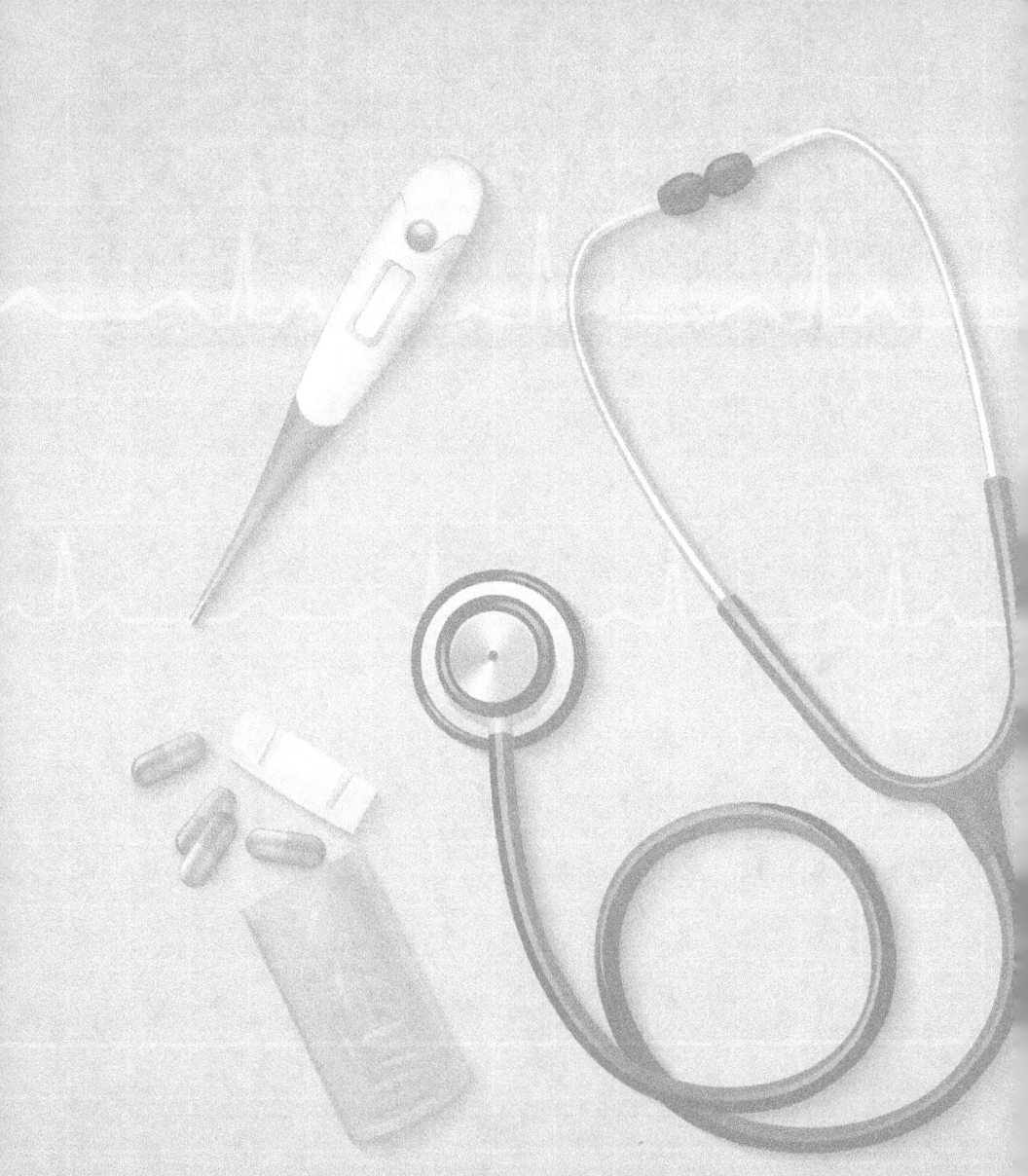

13.1 What does a Journal Editor Look For?

Every manuscript submitted to a journal is evaluated by the journal's editors based on four criteria: scope, quality, innovation, and importance. Analyze your work using these four categories before submitting it for publication. Because this book is about writing your paper, my advice is to make it as simple for a reader (and reviewer) to evaluate your work as possible when they read it.

Write in such a way that it is clear what your work is about, what is new and how it is related to previously published work, and why it is important. Also, ensure that your language is of sufficient quality so that the reader can accurately assess the scientific quality.

13.2 Scope

The most common reason for your manuscript being rejected is that you submitted it to the wrong journal. If the title of the paper does not correspond to the scope of the journal, the manuscript will be rejected. As a result, you should conduct extensive research on the scope of any publication to which you intend to submit and ensure that the scopes are compatible.

13.3 Quality

The quality of the work being reported, as well as the quality of the reporting which is, the written manuscript, are two important quality dimensions in journal articles. The work's quality is fundamentally a scientific judgment in terms of assessing the results and integrating them into the larger context of the scientific field.

In other words, you wish the editors, reviewers, and readers to focus on the scientific quality of your work. Readers should be able to understand the language if it is simple (and the opening paragraph should be the easiest). The readers who will understand and evaluate the work will be the journal's editors and reviewers.

13.4 Novelty

The science journal's explicit goal is to add to the corpus of knowledge in the scientific field. As a consequence, a journal paper must contribute to that body of knowledge by introducing new theories, designs, models, methods, data, or analyses. As a result, a thorough review of the literature and extensive citations is required to determine which aspects of the presented work are novel. Of course, not everything in the newspaper needs to be fresh. Publications are frequently compared to progress reports, which are issued when a major milestone in the course of a research project is reached. In this case, some sections of the publication should evaluate previously published work from the same effort.

A good rule of thumb is that at least half of the results must be unique. If more than half of the results you provide have already been published, you have most likely not done enough new work to justify a new publication. Of course, a thorough explanation of what is new is required.

13.5 Significance

The third and most important requirement for publication is that the work should be noteworthy enough. The article's significance should be evaluated through the eyes of the readers: how many people will read it and apply the information to science.

13.6 Choosing the Right Journal

After putting in so much effort to create a flawless article, the next significant challenge is locating the ideal scientific publication to submit the research. Which one will give your study the attention it deserves? Which one will make your work stand out the most? Which is the gold standard in your field of study? Choosing the best journal in which to publish your work may be more difficult than you think.

To determine a journal's influence, use journal metrics.

Cite Score metrics – It assists in determining the importance of journal citations. Scopus, the largest global abstract and citation database of peer-reviewed publications, was used to generate metrics that are free, complete, transparent, and up to date.

SCImago Journal Rank (SJR) – It is based on the idea of transferring prestige between journals via citation links.

Source Normalized Impact per Paper (SNIP) – This is a complicated metric that considers field-specific citation practices.

Journal Impact Factor(JIP) - The Journal Impact Factor is calculated by Clarivate Analytics as the average of citations received in a specified year to a journal's preceding two years of publications divided by the sum of "citable" publications in the preceding two years.

H-index - Despite its origins as an algorithm, the H-index has been used to aggregate higher-order aggregations of research articles, such as journals.

Go to Journal Insights if it is available, to learn more about the journal's impact, speed, and reach. It comprises:

Impact: The average number of citations for a work published in this journal.

Speed: The average duration in weeks it takes to review an item. In other words, the average amount of time it takes an article during the production process to reach major publication milestones.

Reach: Over the last five years, the total number of downloads at the national/international level.

13.7 Avoiding Inappropriate Journal

Regrettably, the open-access publishing model, in which researchers pay for publishing and readers read the papers for free, has given way to a heinous phenomenon: the predatory journal. These are forgeries of scientific publications that proclaim to serve the science world but are primarily concerned with profit. Despite having a legitimate-looking website and a sensible name, these journals are not legitimate. They almost never read papers, accept any paper submitted after a sham peer review, and then charge authors money to have their work published on a website. Publishing a scientific work in a predatory magazine is more than just a waste of money; it is a blemish on the author's notoriety and a stumbling block to the author's career.

To avoid predatory journals, ask yourself the following questions before submitting an article to one you've never heard of):

- Do you or any of your coworkers know anything about the journal?
- Is it easy to find the contact details of the publisher?

- Is it possible to get in touch with the publisher by phone, email, or mail?
- Is the journal's method of peer review specified?
- Have you previously read any of the journal's articles?
- Are any of the services you use indexing articles?
- Is it simple to locate the journal's most recent publications?
- Are you aware of any of the editorial board members?
- Is it clear how much money you'll need to pay?
- Is there any information on the journal's website about the purpose of these fees and when they will be implemented?

13.8 Avoiding Double Publications

Peer-reviewed journals almost don't recommend double publication. It is the practice of submitting a manuscript for publication that is nearly identical to one that was previously published in any other journal). Double submission is an illegal act in which the same or nearly identical work is considered for publication by two journals at the same time.

While it is obvious not to submit a previously published paper, it is not always easy to tell when duplicate content crosses the line into duplicate publication.

13.9 Conclusions

Unfortunately, double publication is a problem that journal editors must occasionally deal with. Occasionally, the problem arises unintentionally as a result of poor citations and a failure to consider the situation. Authors frequently try to inflate their publication counts by disseminating their work thinly to make it to too many papers. After the authors learn the techniques, the editors will face fewer and fewer challenges.

14

FURTHER READING

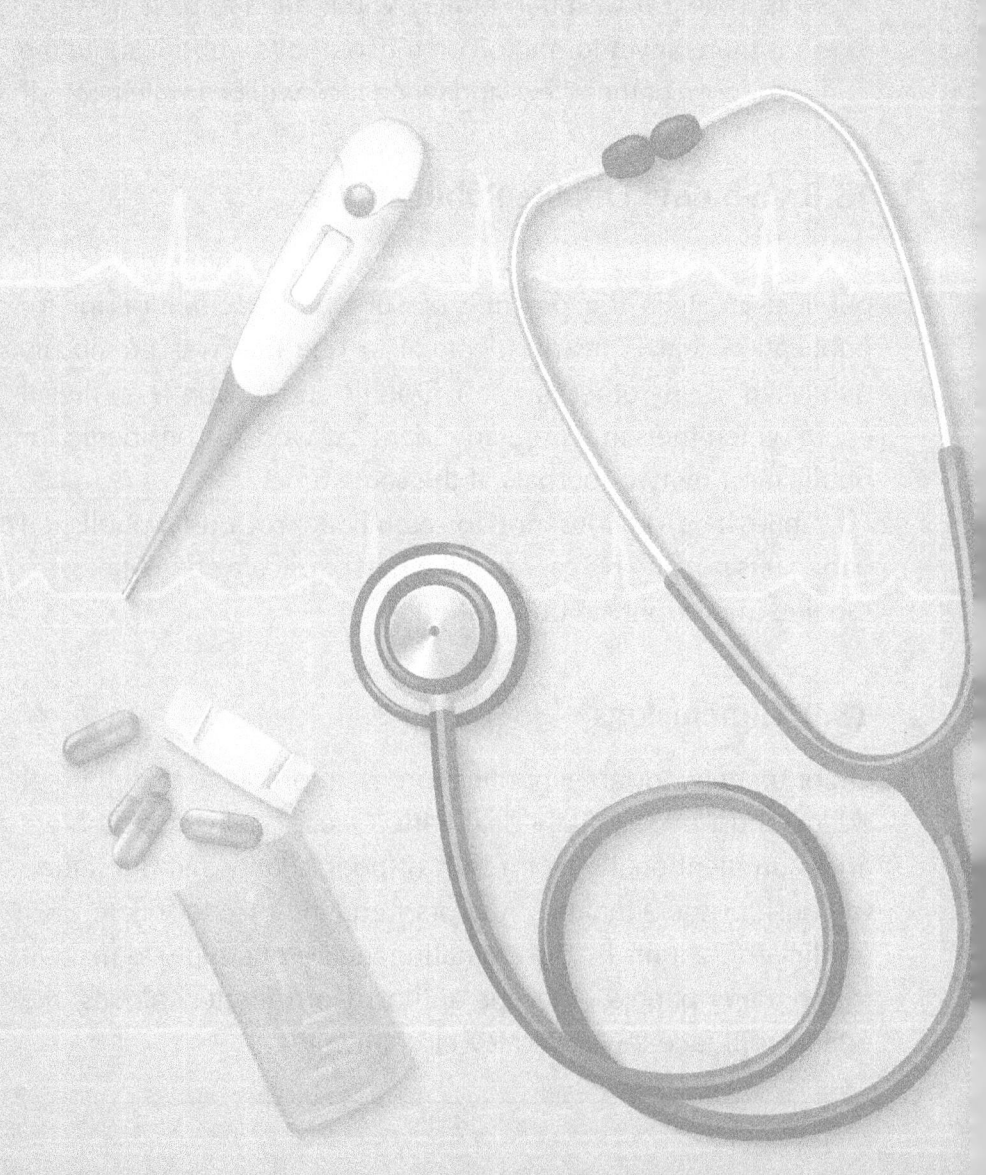

1. Essentials of Writing Biomedical Research Papers. Mimi Zeiger. 2nd Edition. McGraw Hill Professional

2. What Every Medical Writer Needs to Know. Robert B. Taylor. Springer.

3. Successful Scientific Writing: A Step-by-Step Guide for the Biological and Medical Sciences, Matthews and Matthews. 4th Edition.

4. Guidebook to Better Medical Writing. Robert L. Iles

5. On Writing Well: The Classic Guide to Writing Nonfiction, William Zinsser, 30th Anniversary edition.

6. The Elements of Style. William Strunk Jr., E.B. White

7. Sin and Syntax, Constance Hale.

8. Sackett DL et al. (2000) Evidence-based Medicine How to Practice and Teach EBM. London: Churchill Livingstone

9. Strunk and White's classic, The Elements of Style, http://www.bartleby.com/141/.

10. Friedman GD. Be kind to your reader. 1990 Oct;132(4):591-3. Am J Epidemiol

11. Uniform Requirements for Manuscripts Submitted to Biomedical Journals: www.icmje.org

12. Greenhalgh T (2000) How to Read a Paper: the Basics of Evidence-based Medicine. London: Blackwell Medicine Books

13. Elwood JM (1998) Critical Appraisal of Epidemiological Studies and Clinical Trials (2nd Edn). Oxford: Oxford University Press

14. Crombie IK (1996) The Pocket Guide to Critical Appraisal: a Handbook for Health Care Professionals. London: Blackwell Medicine Publishing Group

15. Hill A and Spittlehouse C (2001) What is critical appraisal? Evidence-based Medicine 3: 1–8 [www.evidence-based-medicine.co.uk]
16. Guyatt G and Rennie D (Eds; 2002) Users' Guides to the Medical Literature: a Manual for Evidence-based Clinical Practice. Chicago: American Medical Association
17. Denzin NK, Lincoln YS, eds. Handbook of qualitative research. London: Sage Publications, 1994.